Conversations
with a Dying Friend

John Carmody

PAULIST PRESS
New York/Mahwah

In Memory of Bill Bell,

and for Rita Bell

Book design by Margaret Antonini

Library of Congress Cataloging-in-Publication Data

Carmody, John, 1939–
    Conversations with a dying friend/John Carmody.
      p.   cm.
    ISBN 0-8091-3173-0
    1. Death—Religious aspects—Christianity. 2. Friendship—
Religious aspects—Christianity. 3. Terminal care—Religious
aspects—Christianity. 4. Terminally ill—Religious life.
I. Title.
BT825.C385 1992
236'.1—dc20

                                 92-19560
                                    CIP

Published by Paulist Press
997 Macarthur Boulevard
Mahwah, New Jersey 07430

Printed and bound in the United States of America

Contents

	Preface	v
Chapter One	Shock	1
Chapter Two	Fear	19
Chapter Three	Pain	36
Chapter Four	Wisdom	54
Chapter Five	Love	72

Preface

ॐ

This book is a work of imagination, but I wish it were less real. During the past two years I have watched the struggles of five people with cancer. Several have been close friends, one is a relative, and the others have been colleagues. At this writing two have died, one is near death, one has undergone a third operation, and one has recovered well from a first operation. Each story of course is unique, but the convergence of so many threats has brought death to my consciousness as never before.

In several cases I have spoken at some length with these people, usually either in the hospital or at lunch. Much more frequently, however, they have spoken in the depths of my mind, as I hovered on the verge of sleep or tried to focus on God during morning prayer. The "conversations" presented here derive from both actual discussions and exchanges that only occurred in my mind. Moreover, I have mixed elements from one story with others, and I have thematized the conversations to round out the full measure of what facing death seems to entail. All of the elements on which I focus—shock, fear, pain, wisdom, and love—have been present or needed from the beginning of each story, but I have decided to put them in the sequence that best suggests how the dying people I have known either have or might have used their painful experiences well.

The "Tom" who is my interlocutor is what biblical scholars call a "representative personality," standing for the whole of the other side of the dialogue in which I have been engaged with the several different partners. "John" is I, myself.

Finally, it bears noting not only that I myself have never contracted a serious illness, and so in a significant way don't know what I am talking about, but also that the only response I have found radical enough to match the questions posed by fatal illness is the cross (and resurrection) of Christ. At the same time, I have wanted to flee pious language like the plague, lest it disfigure or abuse the experiences of the people who have been haunting my mind. Others will have to judge how well I have succeeded and whether these conversations carry any of the genuine comfort of Christ. My thanks to the friends who have not hidden their pains are like the thanks of an apprentice to a master. If any good comes from this book (if it becomes something one can hand to people shadowed by death without fearing it may do more harm than good), those who have shown me so much courage and faith deserve most of the credit. Eternal rest grant unto them, O Lord, and let perpetual light shine upon them. May they, and all the departed, rest in peace.

In April, 1992, John Carmody was diagnosed as having incurable bone cancer.

1

Shock

If I begin at the beginning of any of the conversations with dying friends that have been playing in my mind, I find or imagine a shock that has later muted itself but has never disappeared. The dying person himself or herself has usually confessed to finding the diagnosis of serious or terminal cancer shocking— something hard to accept as real. And I have found myself wondering repeatedly how it can be that someone obviously, sometimes vigorously, alive is being invaded steadily by death. This shock seems to me a sign of health and sanity. It says that death appears like an intruder, a stranger neither expected nor welcome. Perhaps the very old experience death's knock on the door differently, but all of my friends have been in what should have been their prime years (they have ranged from fifty-three to seventy-three). So a feeling of unreality has hung over our conversations, actual and imagined, and we have regularly shaken our heads at the fact that we found ourselves talking about or constantly being aware of death.

§∾

Tom: "It's good of you to come so regularly. The nurses are wonderful, and the family has been doing well, but I find I

1

can speak more frankly with you. I hope that's all right—seeing you as a professionally religious type, as well as a friend."

John: "It's fine. I want to do whatever you feel like doing on any given day. I think it's wonderful that you can deal with the cancer as a simple fact, but if the day comes when you can't or don't want to, please just say so."

Tom: "Well, it is a fact, though I have to say it still doesn't seem real. I had felt no pain. I thought the bleeding was an irritation or at worst hemorrhoids. When the doctor said he'd have to operate, I hoped for the best. To find that the case was the worst possible—not only was there cancer but it had spread widely—was a great shock. But still there's no pain, though of course there was the pain of the surgery and the nausea and discomfort of the chemotherapy. Strange. The silence of the cancer is both a comfort and an added burden. I can start to think the whole business is just a dream from which I'll soon wake, but I never do."

John: "You've said that usually you don't feel afraid. Has that continued to be true?"

Tom: "Yes. Maybe it's because there hasn't been much pain. Or because I still haven't *felt* much overflow from the fact that I'm dying. I accept the fact in my mind, but it's still unreal —like a specimen you might pick up on the beach and find interesting but not become engaged with."

John: "I guess that's why we can still talk fairly easily. I don't feel that your sickness has separated you from me—put you across a border into a foreign country. We're still more alike than unlike. I know, mentally, that I'm going to die. I know, by the actuarial tables, that my life is about two-thirds over. But these facts don't mean much emotionally. Death still stands at a distance. Whether deliberately or through a kind of courtesy you may not even appreciate you're showing me, you convey the idea that we share this detachment from death.

We're still both people so alive that death seems foreign. Do you think that will change soon?"

Tom: "I suspect it will. I've already found myself looking at the nurses or visitors as though they should be different from what I see. I remember going to a dinner party shortly after we got the diagnosis. It was something it seemed easier simply to go ahead with than to cancel. I didn't want to tell the people the news we'd just gotten, so Audrey and I tried to behave as though nothing had happened. It was good therapy, actually, because most of the evening I forgot about cancer and death and everything being up for grabs and just enjoyed some ordinary, social conversation. The few times I remembered the real situation I wondered what these people would think, were I to tell them, but I wasn't ready to do that, and it even seemed that to tell them might be cruel."

John: "Is it a great burden, having to wonder about how people will react when they learn you are dying, or having to wonder what they are thinking?"

Tom: "Yes, it can be. On bad days you can feel like a curiosity. I don't blame most people. I remember how I used to feel about people, when I'd learned they had cancer or had suffered a heart attack. There's a prurience hanging around death, waiting to lure us in. And sometimes I used to feel a whole welter of emotions: fortunate, for being healthy; superior, maybe, though obviously for no good reason; even guilty, to have been spared such a test, perhaps because I wasn't ready for it. I remember reading novels about war and thinking that having to face death probably is the crisis that makes us mature. So I think it's likely that meeting someone they know is dying is going to shake many people up. Again, the elderly seem to handle this better than the rest of us, as though reading the obituaries of classmates, and going to funerals, and just seeing their friends removed one by one makes death part and parcel of their lives. But people my age are still avoiding death, because they still can. I bear them the bad news that their time of avoidance is lessening."

John: "I have to say that talking with you, following the course of your illness, certainly has made me more sober. In fact, it's made me grateful to you, in perhaps a perverse way, because I've had to think hard about what should be important to me. Yes, you're some years older than I, but not so many that I can't imagine myself getting the news you've gotten some day not too far from now. I guess the most consoling thing is that I don't find myself with any great regrets, and I'm sure that your feeling that way, your having no great regrets, has helped me immensely. I remember the day you said that, yes, there were projects you'd like to complete and trips you'd like to take, but that they weren't really very important. To be able to say that has become one of my main goals. You see, I'm making you my teacher or model—that should embarrass you properly!"

Tom: "Indeed it should. If I thought you were fully serious, I might get worried, but I think I know what you mean. That's another tricky issue: how much to try, deliberately, to let others benefit from my experience. I guess I've been reluctant to face how complicated that question is. My general impression, which I don't think is overly cynical, is that people only learn what they are ready to learn. If somebody is ready to take stock, reconsider priorities, face the fact that life is short, then maybe dealing with me will be helpful. If not, I doubt that my cancer, or his father's heart attack, or her mother's senility is going to make much of an impact. Certainly I kept myself well guarded against premature thoughts of death for many years. I was too busy with plans and ambitions. So I don't expect most people to have their lives changed greatly by dealing with me or any other terminal patient. Yet, maybe I have to be ready to make a difference, if someone does show a susceptibility. What, though, should I try to teach such a person? That's another huge issue.

You don't want people becoming morbid. Young people, especially, need the sort of drive that often depends on tunnel vision, animal vigor, seizing the day."

John: "True, yet you may be underestimating your own significance. At least with your friends, you've got a reputation for honesty and realism. When they find that you're as honest in dealing with your cancer as you were with your contracts or your kids' emotional problems, they're impressed. They've told me that. In fact, I think they're more than impressed. They're pleased—that someone is staying consistent to the end, practicing what he preached. Indeed, it may be that death is giving you a chance to show that honesty can be the best policy right to the end. We all sense that a lot of the attitudes our culture assumes toward death, or illness, or failure are dishonest, even cowardly. When you cut through all that and insist on being yourself, it's a victory for fresh air."

§∞

Tom: "I've been thinking about what you said yesterday about honesty. You know, even the doctors waffle about my condition. Hinson is a straight shooter, almost too much so, in fact, as though truth were a monkey he had to get off his back. Bracken only gets to the bottom line if I push him. He'd rather talk about experimental therapies or ways to make me more comfortable. Audrey has been wonderful, knowing precisely when I wanted to speak brutally honestly and when I wanted to drop the bottom line for a while and just enjoy the moment. In many ways it's harder on her than on me, of course. And that, in turn, means that I feel more worry and regret and even guilt about her than about myself. Very strange. All the ties of marriage get intensified. If you've become used to living as much for the other person as for yourself, your dying becomes common property."

John: "Yes, I've watched Audrey quite closely, wondering, to be honest, whether your assurances that she is very strong were valid. I've been very impressed. You two do know one another very well. I also think that it's another sign of your mental or spiritual health that you haven't let the cancer narrow you in upon yourself. I remember a friend of mine complaining, with a rueful laugh, that the worst effect of his bad back was the self-concern (he was a psychological type, so he called it 'narcissism') it generated. But it must be hard at times. You must sometimes feel alone."

Tom: "Oh yes. Especially at night, when everyone's gone and it's deathly quiet, to coin a phrase. It comes home to me then that no one can do this dying but me. I've got to face it, or accept it, by myself. Not that I'm not grateful for the concern, the prayers, the interest that other people show. But at the end it will be just me, going through something no one else can explain or describe from experience. Funny, isn't it, that the most crucial bit of advice we'd like to have available can't be. People have been dying for tens of thousands of years, yet every one of us faces it afresh, like a novice or a virgin."

John: "I've thought about that too. It has its parallels with education: each generation has to make the same mistakes, it seems, verifying the old saw, 'You can't put old heads on young shoulders.' But certainly death is the most extreme case. When I think as a theologian, though, something interesting comes to mind. Saint Paul talks about living and dying with Christ, and such talk gets taken into the symbolism for baptism, as you know. I suspect that for Paul something very physical, if still mystical, was at work. He so identified himself with Christ that the death of Christ framed his expectations. What had happened to Christ, he thought, had to happen to him if he was to reap the full fruits of his faith. Dying was the passageway, the passover, to wherever or whoever Christ now was. Does that make any sense to you?"

Tom: "Only a little. I was going to ask you what they taught you in the seminary about death. What did they say would happen? Even as I ask you, though, the same question comes to mind: Who could know? Who's actually been there?"

John: "Oh they didn't have a lot to say. All of the 'four last things' (death, judgment, heaven and hell) were very mysterious, and the better teachers and books owned up to that completely. I've told you before about Karl Rahner, my favorite theologian during seminary days—the one who kept me sane. Rahner speaks of all the cautions that should attend any assertions about the last things, arguing that what we find in scripture, the creeds, and the rest of the Christian tradition are only symbols hinting at the mysteriousness of what it means to be saved into God. He thinks these symbols are precious beyond compare, but he's dead-set against the literalism you find in some fundamentalists, who think of the book of Revelation as a series of snapshots of what heaven is like—the 144,000, the plagues, the riders, all the rest. Anyway, Rahner's main instinct is that death may give us the chance to do something we've wanted to do all our lives but have never been able to accomplish: sum ourselves up, say yes or no definitively."

Tom: "Say yes or no to what?"

John: "To God, to our lives, to the selves we've become. Before death we're always distracted and we can't know what we really think or who we really want to be. Rahner imagines that death suspends the whirl of our thoughts and emotions, cuts through all the dividedness of our conscience, and lets us see what's really been at stake."

Tom: "What's really been at stake, in his view?"

John: "Ah, you keep pushing me. I wish I were a better Rahnerian. I think what he or at least I think has really been at stake is freely accepting, in fact loving, what has had to be in our lives, their necessity. I mean all the things we didn't choose or have any say about and yet shaped so much of our lives: who our parents were, how they treated us, when and where we grew up, who happened to cross our path and influence us, what kind of health we had, what kind of intelligence we were given, and on and on. Certainly we all have to make significant choices, and so it's very important to discover the freedom we possess. But so much in our lives is out of our control that saying yes to God must mean accepting from God all the constraints and influences about which we had no say. In a way, we even have to forgive God for having made us so imperfect or placed us in less than ideal circumstances. Maybe that's a lot of what goes on when we meet God at death. Maybe we say yes to God, as much as we can, and ask God to say yes to us—to accept us, despite all our sins and defects."

Tom: "Interesting. You're saying that imperfection, the messiness of life, is something we have to forgive God for making. Does that include my cancer?"

John: "I think so. This is all very difficult stuff, you know, getting into problems that any sane theologian stays far away from: providence, how God's will relates to human freedom, how God moves in the natural world. But I think that we finally have to give God a blank check. You know the line from the book of Job, 'Though he slay me, yet will I trust him.' I've heard people condemn the God described in the book of Job as immoral (he plays with Job, he kills Job's children). Yet that's not the point. The point is that Job is right both to protest the injustice he thinks he sees in the world and finally to bow his head in submission: he was not there when God ordered the world in the beginning; he doesn't, can't, know the full proportions of God's plan. So he has to trust God—force God, by trusting him—to be just and good. I think we all have to do this. There's a sense in which God is responsible for your cancer. Who else made the universe in which your cancer occurs as one of the myriad actualizations of the even more myriad interactions among all the atoms and molecules? That doesn't mean I'm ok, you're ok, cancer's ok—because God's ok. Obviously your cancer is terrible: a disorder, something that should not be. And yet, and yet—it's ultimately something that God chose when God decided to make this given universe in which you and I exist. So even though we have to die, sometimes prematurely, it may be that God has purposes for our death, and so for the cancer or heart disease or accident that caused it, beyond our reckoning. I know that cancer, or even more the results of human evil, such as the holocaust, cause some people, perhaps many people, to reject the idea of a good God. But I think such a rejection is premature. We just can't know the overall tally sheet about the universe. We just can't say that God isn't weaving both physical evils and moral evils into something comprehensive that will not only manifest the goodness of God but will even prove to have served our passage to complete happiness with God in heaven. And, as Christians, we have to reckon with the fact that God did not spare his own Son the consequences of an imperfect world but allowed, in a sense chose, that Jesus had to hang from the cross and die as a victim of human malice."

$\gtrsim$

John: "Well, how's the great man today? Are your spirits holding up?"

Tom: "Pretty well, though I found the weekend depressing. All the rain didn't help, and Nancy, my youngest daughter —have you met her? She's been away at college—fell apart. Poor kid. She's been daddy's little girl all her life, and now daddy is walking out on her."

John: "Poor thing. My sister was somewhat like that when our dad died. She kept hoping for a turn-around, right up to the end. I've often thought she experienced his death much more profoundly than I, because she didn't shield herself so well. She kept letting herself hope. I've always been more stoic."

Tom: "As am I. I guess it's part of the male mystique: give me the facts, and I'll put up with them. By the way, have you heard about Horace Carson? He's been proclaiming himself cured of lung cancer. That doesn't happen very often, you know."

John: "I know. You used to be close to him. What do you think's going on?"

Tom: "Oh I suspect he's scared and has decided to try positive thinking. He's such a public figure that he's always had to keep up appearances. Maybe appearances have started to substitute for reality. They say that he still looks pretty good, though he wheezes badly. Crazy—he won't even stop smoking."

John: "Wow. That is crazy. Poor man. You know, he's always seemed to me somewhat haunted. People say that in the old days he was a model of self-confidence, but in the time I've known him he's been terribly nervous. His eyes are always moving and he can't keep still. But I've never made more than social conversation with him, chit-chat about sports or city politics."

Tom: "Tell me more about accepting death as part of a bigger picture. I find that comforting, somehow, and it seems to me that getting a hold on what death might mean, in a bigger picture, is half the battle of coping with it. Horace, I suspect, keeps running precisely because he has no way of making cancer or death meaningful."

John: "Well, where do we get our bigger pictures? That's one of the most basic questions, I guess. Traditionally people's religions, which were simply the foundational beliefs of their whole culture, offered them myths and rituals that somewhat tamed death by making it the concluding part of a life-cycle filled with initiations into deeper meaning. Death, then, could be seen as simply the final, most mysterious of these initiations. That sort of culture has broken apart for us in the modern west. Yet Christian faith continues to say that whether we live or die we belong to God. That's the bigger picture I find most consoling: we belong to God. We did not make ourselves, so we don't have to supply all our meaning or value. Just as we have to trust that there is a God, a maker, and that God gives our lives great meaning, so we have to trust that God will see us through death. Certainly there are other perspectives, other ways of speaking about a bigger picture, but I am most drawn to one that makes death something very personal between us and God."

Tom: "As you know, much of the religion that I was taught was pretty raw: sinners going to hell, the just going to heaven, 'sin' and 'justice' or 'virtue' quite black and white. I gave that up by the time I was in high school. I've gone to church since early in our marriage, but I've never bothered much with the doctrines. I couldn't seem to get my mind around them, though probably I didn't try very hard. But I did find the ceremonies and the fellowship comforting. After a while they became a habit, so I missed them if I was sick or we were traveling. Now I believe or hope that at death I will enter into something greater than myself, but I don't have a clear idea of what that might mean, nor of how it relates to Christ."

John: "Well, how much do you want me to say? I think God is present in any experience or symbol that helps us get through our days, or perhaps even more our nights, so if you're content with the idea of passing over into God, maybe that should be enough."

Tom: "No. I'm content, but I know there's more to be said. So, if you're willing, I'd like to hear it."

John: "I'm willing enough. The question is how able I am. Let's go right for the jugular. The creed emphasizes that the life and death of Christ were 'for us men (human beings, we'd say nowadays) and our salvation.' The root meaning of 'salvation' revolves around health or making-healthy. So, the idea is that what Jesus said, did, was, and suffered can be, should be, a way for us to be healed of our brokenness, relieved of our ignorance and misery, made whole, as all along we've wanted to be. How can faith in Jesus and Jesus' God make us whole? A very large question. I think the crux of it, though, is that when one focuses on the death and resurrection of Jesus as the capstone of his life, nearly incredible possibilities open. The death that is the greatest threat to our wholeness, to the meaningfulness of our existence, may not be the final word—because Jesus escaped from death, triumphed over death. The evil that can make life seem useless may not be the final word—because the goodness of Jesus, his love, proved stronger. The evil done to him did not destroy him, if God raised him from the dead and put a seal, a stamp of ratification, on his teaching and example. All of which leads me to say, gingerly (because we're dealing with matters of faith, not hard facts or arguable theories), that at death the something greater we enter into is the mystery of Christ, now freed of the limitations that either the humanity of Jesus or our own humanity necessarily places upon it. Saint Paul, again, speaks of the 'body' of Christ, which he considers to be a living, organic whole. Between Christ and those who believe in Christ there is a bond, a unity, such that the fate of one makes an impact on the fate of the other. Saint John seems to be saying the same thing, with his figure of the vine and the branches. I don't mean to give you a disquisition on biblical theology, but when I start to stammer about what faith says we enter at death, these are the ideas that come to mind. According to Paul and John, death 'merely' consummates the connections or identification that faith had given us to God and Christ while we were living. This 'connection' of course is hard to pin down. But I think it can build on a sense many people develop that their lives are part of a much greater process, and that their deaths may complete at least one phase of their participation in such a greater process. Christians, then, would simply claim to be specifying or deepening something that all sorts of people have felt throughout history. And this would tie in with the notion that God has always given people—all people—sufficient grace for salvation."

Tom: "So, Christian faith is not something completely unique or set apart from the experience of people who aren't Christians."

John: "Right. Christian faith reveals or clarifies how God is at work in all people's lives."

Tom: "What, then, is the special value of Jesus or Christian faith? Aren't you saying that people can accomplish the essentials of their lives, of what God asks of them, even if they haven't formally committed themselves to Christ?"

John: "Yes, I am saying that. But think a bit about the value of having formal commitments, explicit creeds, symbols and models that claim to reveal what God is doing everywhere. Isn't it great progress to have a theory of cancer that clarifies what has been going on in the millions of people who have suffered and died from cancer through the centuries? Doesn't it tame cancer a lot just to know what it is and how it operates? And, of course, with such knowledge comes the possibility of curing cancer. Sure, things are less physical and certain when we're in the realm of faith, God, and ultimate meaning. But if our beliefs and symbols are true—if Jesus really has revealed crucial aspects of the character of God, and so of the character of human existence—then we're wonderfully enriched. The problem, I think, has not been that Christians haven't had a wonderful message to proclaim, but that too often we've lost the mysteriousness that gives what we proclaim its full resonance and gives us great reason to be very humble when we talk about how salvation, or the grace of God, or anything else like that actually works out in people's lives."

ഔ

Tom: "Yesterday one of the nurses asked me who you were and what we were talking about. 'It sounds terribly serious,' she said. I had to laugh. I guess it does sound terribly serious. Do you talk this way with all the people you visit in the hospital?"

John: "Hardly. Part of the joy of coming to see you is that you are so open about your condition, and another part is that you want to probe the implications for faith. That's a rare combination."

Tom: "Why? I would think most people seriously ill would want to get all the help they could to understand the implications of what was happening to them. As soon as I say that, though, I realize that most of the time I've visited people in the hospital it's been pretty awkward."

John: "I really don't know why it's so hard for people to speak simply yet deeply about what is most important to them —even when they're facing death. If pressed I'd say that talking about God and faith and salvation might make them nervous, because it can conjure up judgment and guilt, but then I reflect that most healthy people I meet don't speak comfortably about anything I would consider serious or profound, so maybe it's more a matter of sick people simply continuing with patterns they established when they were well. If you look at our general American culture with a contemplative eye, searching for signs that people want to know about meaning and stupidity, life and death, you come away disappointed most of the time."

Tom: "You know, one of the good things about being sick, if you can call anything about it good, has been the way it's freed me of so many petty concerns. I simply couldn't care less now what the stock market is doing or who's gaining power at city hall. Part of me thinks that isn't completely right: Shouldn't I stay interested in life and people right to the end? But another part, rooted in the fatigue growing in my body, says: 'Forget it. It never was very important.' On the other hand, I have quite an appetite for the kind of questions you and I have been discussing. My spirit, you might say, has been profiting from the weakness of my body and the obvious fact that very soon I'm not going to have any position in the stock market or any concern with city hall."

John: "Some of the old meditation masters we had to read in the seminary used to propose an exercise to make their readers serious about the religious life. 'Suppose you learned that you were going to die in a month,' they would say. 'What would you want to have done with your life?' The obvious point was to get you to say that you'd want to have concerned yourself more with pleasing God, before whom you would soon appear to be judged. Well, that all sounds too much focused on fear to be fully satisfying nowadays, when people rightly hear more about the love of God and God's desire that we use our freedom creatively. On the other hand, to be serious about one's life, even to worry about what one has become and what one has failed to accomplish—that seems to be one of the marks of a mature person. Often there's not much we can do about the past, except to repent of our failings and pledge not to repeat them in the future. But unless we're interested in what we have become, and are concerned about what we should be becoming in the future, we're not very serious or impressive people. Does that make sense to you, or am I just reflecting years of admiration for Kierkegaard and others who have spoken eloquently about what it takes to become a significant self?"

Tom: "No, it make good sense. I've never felt I had very

good tools for handling the question of what I should be aiming to become in my life, but I've always been bothered by people who were only interested in money, or possessions, or news. The older I got, the less I looked forward to evenings out, because so often they turned out to be trivial. I came to prefer staying home with a good book or listening to good music. I came to love simply thinking about what had happened during the day and trying to get it in perspective. I think that's served me well in the hospital. Thinking about the significance of what was happening to me wasn't novel. I didn't have to begin from scratch."

John: "I suppose you know about the examination of conscience: taking stock of one's actions and thoughts before God on a regular basis. Some of the most helpful spiritual writing I read years ago showed how the examination could become a way to pray. The idea is to move from the review of one's behavior or thoughts to the God—the mysterious blank, or maybe an image of Christ—in whose presence one has been making the review. It is more important, most good writers on prayer say, to linger with God, talk with God, give one's whole being over to God than to focus on the particulars of one's day, yet by beginning with such particulars one's prayer to God gets a solid footing, a toehold in the real world."

Tom: "So you're saying that we can take reflection and make it prayerful, simply by doing it in the presence of God."

John: "Right. And the more what we reflect upon becomes a stimulus to talk about our lives with God, or simply to be with God wordlessly, the more prayerful the reflection."

Tom: "But what is this 'presence' of God you mentioned? I've heard it frequently through the years, but I never could get a clear picture of what it meant."

John: "I don't think there is a clear picture, because God isn't something we can get our minds around. Many people rightly prefer to speak with Jesus, Mary, or one of the saints, precisely because we can get our minds around them. But God is something like the air: hard to notice in itself, more a medium of vision than something to focus upon. Some theologians say that God is the 'horizon' against which we do all our thinking. You know how a bright idea seems to pop up or step out from a formless background. That background is God, in the sense that everything particular or definite depends on the whole to set it off and God is the whole. Anyway, the point is that when one examines one's conscience 'in the presence of God' one simply projects or points one's mind and heart toward the blank mystery of the whole (or, as I've said, toward a picture of Christ). Then a third dimension or a second party comes into the equation. We aren't reflecting alone. We're sharing our thoughts, our regrets, our hopes, our loves. And sometimes it can strike us that we're never really alone, even when we're not paying attention to this third dimension or second party. Whenever we do pay attention it is there, so it must be there all the time, because we could pay attention, in theory, anytime. We're never alone—isn't that provocative?"

Tom: "It seems pretty mystical to me, but what do I know? I'm more drawn to the idea that by thinking about my situation with some desire to share my thoughts with God I may be praying, which presumably would please God."

John: "Presumably, inasmuch as prayer is essentially just trying to love and commune with God. If the gospels teach us anything, it is that God desires our love, in response to the love God has lavished upon us. It's taken me a long time to personalize this, since, like most people, I don't think of myself as anything that would hold much intrigue for God. But the more I try to make sense of the message of Jesus, the more it seems clear that God greatly desires us human beings, and that God's desire for us—God's ardent wish that we open up and love him back—is the real foundation or ground of our significance. If God didn't want us, we wouldn't exist. And if God does want us, like a lover, then our existence must be extraordinary, a true marvel."

2

Fear

Tom: "Last night I became afraid, for the first time in many weeks, and the unnatural, threatening character of this cancer assaulted me. I don't know why this happened. Sometimes I've woken from frightful dreams, but since I got over the initial shock of being diagnosed as having widespread cancer, I haven't feared or even worried very much during my waking hours."

John: "What did you seem to be afraid of?"

Tom: "I'm not sure—dissolving, falling apart, losing the only kind of existence I've ever known. I felt some guilt that I hadn't led a better life, and some regret that I was putting my family and friends through worry and upset. But a lot of it wasn't rational. I just shook at the realization that I was going to die, and that it might be painful."

John: "Well, I'm no psychiatrist, but that seems to me pretty normal or healthy. I suspect it takes some time for the body to get its message through to the brain. And frequently the medium the body uses is the emotions. We've already spoken of the difference between acknowledging something and feeling its full impact. I imagine that much of the natural process the whole human being, body and spirit, goes through on the way to becoming reconciled to death—not just death in the abstract, as a general human necessity, but the quite different matter of one's own very specific death—will usually involve coping with the fear of the unknown and the perhaps painful realities that such a death may entail."

Tom: "People have told me that they, or others they have known, have reacted to the news that they have cancer by thinking, 'Why me? What have I done wrong?' I've only felt that or thought that a little bit. Maybe I would have felt it more had I been younger. But at sixty I'd already seen many friends die and realized I'd been fortunate to survive them. On the other hand, getting the diagnosis did make me wonder whether I had done something wrong—not eaten correctly or had the right mental attitude. There are all sorts of theories flying around about the mental side of cancer, many of them quite loony, but they do make you wonder about what went wrong, why your cells started misbehaving."

John: "Since we're in the area, let me ask you about anger. Have you felt angry that you took ill, were unfairly struck down?"

Tom: "Not very much. My main feeling has been that it's unreal—that I don't know why it happened and I can't determine what it means."

John: "What could it mean that would be frightening?"

Tom: "Well, apart from the loss of identity I mentioned and the prospect of pain, it could mean I've blown it. I've done a lot in my life, and maybe accomplished some good, but I certainly haven't put my life together the way I had hoped. I guess I looked forward to retirement and older age as a time to reflect and make sense of the whole. Nothing cosmic. No burning desire to write a great book to enlighten the world. Just a chance to detach myself from work, family problems, and all the other things that have preoccupied me, so that I could get a better hold on what it's all been about. Perhaps it's foolish to regret not having had that opportunity, and perhaps I never would have come to any satisfying conclusions, but I feel uneasy because I don't know how to finish up or round things off. It's as though they called for the end of the play when I'd only learned my lines through the second act."

John: "Very interesting. I like the desire you have to make sense of the whole. It seems to me very religious, in the best of senses. You know how much nonsense religion attracts or generates, all the bad uses to which it's put. But when we talk about making sense of the whole, or finding how to accept death as a good consummation of one's life, religion can come into its own. The fact is that none of us has ever seen God (bracketing some questions about Jesus, Mary, and the saints). The bottom line of the human condition seems to be that we don't know the most basic things about our situation: where we came from, where we are going, how we stand before God, if there is a God. So we're all even, radically equal, when it comes to death. You've probably seen those medieval depictions of the dance of death, where the pope is hand in hand with a peasant or a blacksmith or a maid. Death is the great leveler. At one time, after they had elected a new pope, someone would go before him in the procession chanting that he was to remember that he had come from dust and unto dust he would return. The signing with ashes on Ash Wednesday, to begin Lent, uses the same symbolism. Anyway, it seems to me that religion does some of its best work when it makes this basic mysteriousness of our human condition a source of wisdom, compassion, and even love. If we can embrace our ignorance, we can push away from all the know-it-alls who keep oppressing or distracting us and finally listen to the silence that is so much more eloquent. In this context, the great service of Jesus and Christian faith would be the encouragement they offer us to brave that silence, face our ignorance, and test the proposition that God will make it nourishing for us."

Tom: "What do you mean, 'make it nourishing for us'? I've got a glimmer, but it's not very strong."

John: "Well, go back to what you said about becoming disgusted with or put off by the trivial conversation that prevails on most social occasions. You said that in recent years you've preferred staying home with a good book or good music and just thinking about the day. Couldn't you say that you found such thinking more nourishing than the chatter of the typical evening out? Couldn't you say that, parallel to the way that a good meal leaves a feeling of contentment, of things being right with your body, a good book or good music or quiet thought about serious matters often leaves a feeling of things being or becoming right with your spirit? The key signs of a right spirit, according to the tradition of the discernment of spirits, are peace and joy. When we have been brought together, reknit or recollected, by God's Spirit, we feel the tranquillity of order (Augustine's definition of peace) and the joy that nothing material or earthly can give. I don't know how to describe joy in terms of something more primitive or component. It seems to be elemental. Yet most of us have experienced it now and then, usually unexpectedly, and when we do it carries its own warrant. We simply know that for the moment all is right with the world and we have been made to feel this way. Certainly reading a good book doesn't guarantee our being moved to peace and joy, yet often it can take us toward the depths of ourselves, where we can break free of the partial and the distracting to let go and try to float on the mystery of the divine darkness."

Tom: "That's a lot to think about. I gather it comes from your reading in traditional Christian spirituality. But some of it rings true. I have known an extraordinary peace now and then. There have been times when I felt a rush of joy, for what reason I really couldn't say. And this was different from the joy I felt holding my first child, or the joy that falling in love with Audrey brought. Not totally different, by any means. In fact, probably quite alike. Yet not having so clear or obvious a cause. Coming unexpectedly, as though the sunshine, or the rain, had moved the hormones or whatever to create a moment when everything came together perfectly. You're saying that the silence, the mysteriousness, the ignorance, the questions so deep we cannot put them into words—that things like this can nourish the depths or core of our spirits, our selves. You're saying that I might be able to turn the immensity or mystery with which death confronts me into something positive."

John: "Yes. Yes, indeed. I don't want to rush ahead too quickly, or overlook the trials that the darkness of God can carry. But I do want to suggest that what you were looking forward to dealing with in retirement or older age may be with us all the time, only usually we're too busy, too much tied down with other responsibilities, to recognize or deal with it. If I'm right (if the traditional spirituality is right), then the potential blessing of knowing one is going to die fairly soon is the stimulus it may afford us to settle into our depths and experience that we already know something crucial about the darkness that death can spotlight so frighteningly."

§∂

Tom: "Let's go back to the darkness you were talking about. Could a synonym be opaqueness, a sort of cloudiness or obscurity?"

John: "Certainly. One of the great classics on the mysterious presence of God is entitled *The Cloud of Unknowing*. For its author, the presence of the real God is precisely opaque or cloudy."

Tom: "And this all concerns the being of God, what God is in himself?"

John: "Right. In himself, or herself, or itself—all names are inadequate—God is too simple, vast, and ungraspable for our senses or minds. He is bound to seem like the air, as I mentioned, or like a cloud that overshadows the mind, forcing it to stop trying to focus on him as though he were another material thing, or even a clear idea. God invites the mind rather to cede to the heart, to just quiet itself and abide with him, heart to heart."

Tom: "What about the moral side of the darkness or cloudiness? I feel torn or soiled sometimes, as though I could never deal well with a God who expected me to be pure. I have sins of the flesh on my conscience, and sins of the spirit. How can I get rid of these or come to grips with them?"

John: "Good question. It's one thing to get a glimmer of understanding about the way that God is always going to overshadow our minds, because of God's simplicity and infinity, and another thing to realize, to feel to one's marrow, one's unworthiness before God, because God is holy. I think you are fortunate to have brought this moral dimension of your uneasiness—maybe also of your fear?—to explicit awareness. The traditional Christian way of dealing with our sense of unworthiness, our guilt and sin, has been through sacramental confession. Just as we receive the eucharist to be nourished in our life of faith, so we confess our sins in a formal way to be reconciled to God. A lot of unhelpful mystification or fear has sometimes attached itself to sacramental confession or penance, but in itself it is the soul of simplicity and good sense. Human beings need a form through which to express their sorrow for having sinned, acted badly, against other people and even God. It helps us immensely to get out the discontent, the burden on our conscience. Maybe in the perspective of death this can become easier. We have all sinned and fallen short of God's glory, Paul says. We all need to fall on our knees, at least metaphorically, and ask God to accept us despite our selfishness, our lust, our laziness, our hardness toward other people, and all the rest. But if sacramental confession doesn't suit you, because it wasn't part of the tradition in which you were raised, the nearest equivalent might do. That would be simply speaking to God, in your own words, about the things that trouble you and asking God to accept your sorrow, your regrets, as token payment for the redress you wish you could make."

Tom: "Tell me about hell. I hate to admit it, but I've been thinking about hell recently, wondering whether I should be scared."

John: "Umph. Another tough notion. Well, try this. Hell exists, as a symbol, a part of traditional Christian faith, to make clear the seriousness of this venture of making a self in which we are all engaged. Hell says that we can screw things up, badly, even definitively. We can say a final no to God that intends to separate us from God once and for all. In essence, we can refuse to love God, even though loving God is most of what we have been made for. Our freedom is so real, and so important to God, that we can destroy ourselves with it. As the price of creating us with a capacity to engage him in love, God has allowed the possibility that we can disengage ourselves in lovelessness, coldness, self-concern, even hatred—all the varieties of refusing to face the primordial fact of our human condition: we did not make ourselves and don't exist for ourselves. But, after one has said all of this about hell, one can add that we have no certainty that anyone actually exists in hell, definitively separated from God. Because of the way that God has made us, we have to work very hard if we are to frustrate the most basic drive in us, which is to pursue full light and love—God himself. The older Christian view, that the path is narrow and most people do not find it, seems unfair to both God and our actual human nature."

Tom: "But isn't there terrible evil in the world, and don't most of us pay little attention to God, or even to morality, much of our lives?"

John: "Certainly there is terrible evil in the world, and apparently most of us pay little attention to God, or even to morality, much of our lives. Theologians call this the realistic evidence for a doctrine of original sin: something is radically wrong with us. But where sin abounded, Paul again says, grace has abounded the more, and it has never been the Catholic position (here I'm plumping for my own tradition, I guess) that original sin has vitiated human nature. Human nature remains good, though weakened, which would seem to mean that we can trust our basic desires to find God through beauty, truth, justice, service of other people—all the positive inclinations and ambitions we have, which in healthy people tend to outweigh the negative inclinations. Certainly we can be petty, sensual, and hard, but most of us, most of the time, can only be these things with a tinge of awareness that we're denying our better selves. If so, then hell is not our likely destiny. Imperfect as we are, we want to love God, especially if you accept the notion that God is the inmost lure in everything that is noble, beautiful, worth doing, and the like. Most of us are quite weak, but few of us are vicious, energetically evil. Some of us are sick in soul, so afraid or lacking confidence or feeling unlovable that we lash out at others and seem cynical. But even that sort of person, who can be such a burden, doesn't seem a good candidate for hell, a real hater of God. Only the truly spiritual sinners—the cold-blooded murderers, manipulators, drug barons perhaps—approach profound callousness of soul and hatred of God."

Tom: "Isn't it simpler to say that a good God wouldn't put people in hell, eternal torment, and that Jesus preached and revealed a God almost too good to be true? I'm thinking of the story of the prodigal son, which I read the other day and really appreciated for the first time."

John: "Touché. As in so many other cases, the simpler way is indeed the better. When we put aside all the speculation about what constitutes hell and how God deals with those who are confused or sick in spirit, we can come back to the basic stories of the Christian tradition, most of which show God to be precisely as you indicated, almost too good to be believed. Jesus doesn't rail at sinners as much as he goes out to them, saying that God is willing to forgive them, us, seventy times seven. True, Jesus has some harsh words for the hypocrites who hardened their hearts against him, but the greater burden of his teaching is the new opportunity dawning with his presence. The 'kingdom of God' that Jesus talks about is really a time of completely new beginnings. In fact Paul speaks of Christ himself as being a new creation. This newness extends itself in many different directions, but one of the most important has to do with the burdens and patterns established by sin, both individual and social. Individuals need only repent (turn themselves around) and believe in the gospel, the good news that God lives in their midst, full of love for them. And in the church, the Christian community, people ought to be able to see new social patterns, new ways of relating to one another, that challenge the tired old ways of hostility and oppression. 'See how they love one another,' early converts supposedly said, when asked why they had joined the church. If we were to focus on things like this, hell would become properly secondary."

$\sim$

John: "Maybe it's time to discuss the example that Jesus offers for dealing with fear. Traditionally Christians have held that Jesus was sinless, so there was no basis in him for fearing the judgment of God, but the story of his agony in the garden of Gethsemane suggests that he felt all the recoil from pain and death that we associate with a normal human being."

Tom: "Do you think that Jesus felt abandoned on the cross? I've always wondered about those words, 'My God, my God, why have you forsaken me?' There the dread that comes out in the scene of Jesus in Gethsemane seems to come to climax, as though Jesus was tempted to despair."

John: "The early Christians went out of their way to assure themselves and any outsiders to whom they were speaking that Jesus was fully human. Many of the earliest heretics were people who denied not the divinity of Christ but his full humanity. So we can take it as mainstream Christian faith that Jesus was vulnerable in all the ways that having a human body and personality imply. It's hard to know how much to press the accounts given in the New Testament. The authors were telling stories, recalling incidents they had witnessed themselves or others had handed down to them, not writing theological analyses. But they make it clear that Jesus had a full range of emotions—anger, sympathy, love—and that he had to pass through fear and depression to embrace his death. In addition to the healthy reaction of fearing the destruction of himself that death portended, he was depressed that his message and his God had been rejected. On the cross, he quoted from Psalm 22, which begins as a lament ('My God, my God, why have you forsaken me? Why are you so far from helping me, from the words of my groaning?'). The psalm ends with a confession of faith ('People shall tell of the Lord to the coming generation, and proclaim his deliverance to a people yet unborn, that he has wrought it'), but it is not clear whether Jesus meant to call to mind the whole swing of the psalm from depression to faith. Theologians sometimes have said that God never could have abandoned Jesus, inasmuch as Jesus himself was the enfleshment of the divine Son, but that may not be the point. On the cross, Jesus must have suffered terribly. All medical studies of what crucifixion entailed show it was a horrible way to die. Yet most affecting is his sense of having failed or been abandoned. Note, though, what he says at the very end: 'Father, into your hands I commend my spirit.' Jesus lets God be the final depository of everything in his life, even his sense of failure. The lesson would seem to be, in words from the first epistle of John, 'Even when our hearts condemn us, God is greater than our hearts.' "

Tom: "I'm impressed. Jesus went before us in facing death. He learned about death at firsthand, experiencing all of its fears and pains. That's never really come home to me before. Stupid, I guess, not to have reflected on it."

John: "Not stupid. Just never primed, never *having* to see the significance of Jesus' death, because your own death had not yet become fully real."

Tom: "You know, Jesus never has been very real for me. I've liked the stories in the Bible, though some I haven't understood, and I've thought sometimes about the character of Jesus, his personality. But I've never pondered the reason why Jesus should have been born and lived as he did. I've simply accepted what the stories suggest—he was a remarkable man—without getting into the question of God's use of Jesus, God's design in his life."

John: "I think the most touching 'use' God has made of Jesus is to assure us weak, troubled creatures that God knows from the inside what it is like to be human: finite, ignorant, subject to passion and fear and death. The best explanations of Jesus' sinlessness, in my view, make it not something that distances Jesus from the rest of us but something that allowed him to be more human than the rest of us. Jesus was more open to other people, and to God, than the rest of us. He didn't need our defense mechanisms. He wasn't threatened by the mysteriousness of God or the demands of other people the way we tend to be. He could let himself see, feel, and respond. We develop sophisticated strategies for not seeing, not feeling, and not responding, lest we be overwhelmed. But in Jesus God seems to have been spelling out what humanity looks like when it doesn't flee, when it can open itself wide and embrace all of life, the pain and the beauty alike."

Tom: "What means most to me, at this point, is the idea

that I could speak with Jesus, pray to Jesus, as to someone who has gone through what faces me. However commonplace my death, in comparison with Jesus', he and I still share something precious. In the history of Christian piety, have people made a lot of Jesus' sufferings as a reason for thinking he could understand their fears and needs?"

John: "Oh yes. Very much so. The entire medieval period, for complicated reasons, focused on the child Jesus and the man of sorrows hanging on the cross. During the time of the bubonic plague devotion became quite dark and death-centered, sometimes seeming to forget the resurrection of Christ and the Spirit living in believers' hearts."

Tom: "That's another question: how to let myself hope for a resurrection or afterlife. But for the moment let's continue with the suffering Christ. How much did he suffer because of our sins, my sins? Should I feel guilty when I contemplate the cross?"

John: "Well, much Christian piety would say yes, but I think we need to place some qualifications. Theologians have debated whether there would have been an incarnation— whether the Son of God would have taken flesh in the Virgin Mary—had human beings not sinned. The sin they have usually had in mind is the sin of Adam: original sin. We don't know much about original sin. 'Adam' clearly stands for humanity at the beginning, and the sin of Adam stands for the cracks in human nature that seem generic or hereditary, though somewhat culpable in each individual because ratified or worsened by free choice. Many western theologians, including Thomas Aquinas, have thought that had there been no human sin there would not have been an incarnation. The main reason for the Son of God's taking flesh, in their view, was to redeem human beings from sin—repair the damage they had done. One can take other tacks, arguing that revelation and divinization (God's disclosing something of the inner divine nature, and God's giving human beings a share in divine life) would have been good enough reasons for an incarnation, apart from the need to redeem sinful humanity. But for present purposes the point would seem to be that when I approach Christ on the cross I do well to think that Christ died not just for human beings en masse but for each individual, including me. He did this, and the Father 'sent' him, out of love. That love sustained him through his sufferings, enabling him to bear all that he had to bear. Images of oneself banging in the nails or directly causing Christ's pains probably are overheated, but to engage one's own need for redemption, one's own great desire to cast off all that has been wrong and soiled in one's own life, with Christ on the cross would seem very healthy. Not only does Christ represent in spades the mysterious necessity that all of us human beings have to die and most of us have to suffer, he also represents the unthinkable mercy that God has made this necessity into a vehicle that might move us through death into a perfectly fulfilling new life. The love of God, most dramatically shown on the cross, is the force that faith says can defeat death and sin, that is stronger than the worst that is in us—than the worst that is in the universe."

ভ

Tom: "But how do I make these ideas concrete? How can they mediate an encounter with God or Jesus that would help me to feel my kinship or solidarity with Jesus in death?"

John: "Only by making them forms of prayer. Theology has to serve prayer—direct, personal encounter with God—or it remains merely academic. The typical manual of theology has been about as prayerful as a book on auto mechanics."

Tom: "I know something about prayer, actually, though a couple of months ago I would never have claimed to. I have been talking to God about my illness and coming death. Not very well, I'm sure. And often not for myself so much as for my family. Their distress bothers me as much, often more, than my own. Even though I'm the only one who can do this dying, it is affecting them deeply—more deeply than I would ever have thought. My kids seem shaken, though I'm sure they'll finally pull through it fine. But I have been moved to ask God to help them bear my dying and learn from it whatever they should. And of course I've been asking God to help me to bear it and learn what I should. In this praying, I suppose I've depended on certain articles of faith. But they have not been very prominent. It's been enough to believe, or try to believe, in God—a superior power holding the world in his hands. It's been enough to read the New Testament, see how often Jesus is praying or commending prayer, and try to cry out to God as my Father, my helper, my way to make sense of this trial and finally surrender myself: 'Thy will be done.' I can't tell you how grateful I am to have had the Lord's Prayer as a resource since childhood. It comes naturally to my lips, summing up everything I want to say."

John: "That's beautiful—and precisely what religious educators hope will happen, when they drum those prayers into children's heads."

Tom: "But how can I know, or feel, that God is hearing my prayer? What should I expect to happen?"

John: "I don't mean to avoid your question, but I think the first thing one must say is that God, the Holy Spirit (whom Christian tradition tends to make the mover of people's prayers), deals with all of us as individuals. My patterns of prayer may not be yours and probably should not be. Prayer is so personal, so much simply the giving of ourselves over to God and requesting that God give the divine self back to us in return, that it's bound to vary greatly from person to person. Having said that, however, I think one also has to say that many people who pray regularly report that God 'answers' their petitions and love by leaving them somehow quieted, pacified, more integral and resigned, in a good sense, than they were when they began their prayer. If we really are reaching out to God, and not just daydreaming or entertaining an idea of God, prayer is bound to remind us, in some visceral way, that we are not the ones in charge. God is the one in charge. So the realism to which prayer educates us has a lot to do with the priority of God's will. This doesn't mean that we get a vision of what God's will for us will be, in great particularity. Usually it rather means that we realize, for the nth time, that we can never know the plan of which we are only a small part and so must trust that God has good uses for us. More precisely, we must trust that God has good uses for our sufferings and death, bare or even barren though such a trust may sometimes seem."

Tom: "You're back to the blank check again."

John: "Exactly, although with some particulars now to the fore. In prayer that leaves us content, we are letting God write in what God wants, when it comes to cashing out the specific way that we suffer and die and the specific effects our suffering and dying produce. We are trying to say, in our prayer, 'Lord, do something with this mess that I am, that I have so often been. Use me, and so help me to be a profitable servant, despite all the ways I have failed you in the past, all the ways I've wasted my talents and neglected you.' "

Tom: "Do you think that kind of prayer can bring people peace? I think it might. It's the kind of prayer I was groping after."

John: "You'll have to judge that for yourself, but I think and hope so. I stress that you'll have to judge it for yourself because I think it's absolutely crucial not to start thinking one's prayer *ought* to be, or feel, or proceed in such and such a way. Especially, people shouldn't burden themselves with the responsibility of saying pious things, feeling pious thoughts. If pious words genuinely express what's on your mind, wonderful. But if what's on your mind is outrage, anger, hurt, whatever, that's what you should speak out to God. The same with what you are feeling. If you're feeling low, in pain, abandoned, that's what you should bring to God, however mutely or inadequately. Prayer has to be utterly, scathingly honest or it disserves both ourselves and God."

Tom: "I like that. I think that I, and many men, have tended to shy away from prayer because it seemed to require nice phrases and pious feelings we couldn't honestly repeat or feel."

John: "Going back to the question of how God answers our prayers, though, let me add that, when we do deal with God utterly honestly, often we come away strangely comforted, especially when such honest dealing has brought us to confess our wrongness or weakness—our need—and be reminded that Jesus came above all to deal with sinners, the sick, the needy. The great insight of the sixteenth century Protestant reformers was the gratuity of salvation. We don't please God because we have good works, an impressive resume. Rather God takes the initiative and makes us pleasing, saving us—loving us back to wholeness—because of God's own goodness. Justification—being made right with God—comes through faith (opening ourselves to the offer of God's forgiveness and love). When we pray utterly honestly, speaking from the heart about what's troubling us and then listening (holding ourselves attentive in silence) for God's response, we often experience something of such justification, such being moved to a new constellation of our thoughts and emotions or a new stance toward God. I think this frequently is the 'answer' God gives us in prayer. At least, that's the way I have experienced it."

Tom: "Tell me, in this context, how to pray about resurrection or afterlife. What is it reasonable to hope?"

John: "Well, that's the sort of thing God could answer for you, were you to ask him. A good theologian would probably tell you that resurrection is a fundamental article of the Christian creed: 'I believe in the Holy Ghost, the holy catholic church, the communion of saints, the forgiveness of sins, the resurrection of the body, and the life of the world to come.' The resurrection of Jesus was the engine driving the entire New Testament proclamation of the significance of Jesus. In the light of his resurrection, his followers reviewed all that he had said, done, and been, coming away convinced that he was the messiah and unique Son of God. Without the resurrection, Jesus would have been simply another moral hero or striking sage. Because of the resurrection, which we cannot separate from the life and death that it consummated, Jesus became for Christians an unsurpassed revelation of God. The entire gospel of John, for example, meditates on Jesus as the incarnation, the enfleshment, of divine wisdom, which he never could have been taken to be had he not been raised as no one before or after him had. To what was he 'raised'? Immediate communion with God; heaven; the 'right hand' of God; the status he had enjoyed as Son prior to his descent into flesh. On and on the figures go, multiplying so as to suggest complete success, complete fulfillment. We have the right, the duty even, to believe that God holds out for us a share in, a store of, this complete fulfillment. That's what the article in the creed confesses, and the confession is entirely because of Jesus. If we live and die with him, we will be raised with him. That's what we can hope and trust, audacious as it may seem."

3

Pain

John: "You're looking more strained today. Was it a rough night?"

Tom: "Yes, quite rough. I guess the painful stages may be coming."

John: "I'm so sorry. That's lousy."

Tom: "Well, the whole thing is lousy, so I guess I'll just have to get stronger. Let me ask you about pain, what sense you make of it."

John: "I don't make any sense of it. I don't think anyone can. I thought I saw in my father's illness pain working as a purifying force, but I may have been grasping for straws. On the other hand, my father did die a beautiful death, as though he felt released from bondage and discontent. We didn't actually see him die, but when we first saw him after his death, very early on the morning of January 1, his face expressed what I can only call a beautiful repose. He was so frail—less than a hundred pounds—that he seemed transparent. I was reminded of those El Greco saints who seem gaunt, elongated, and luminous. I had to think that he had understood his pain as a way to make up for his failings. He had been a bad alcoholic, which had created deep feelings of guilt. I think he used his pain as a way to assuage such guilt, and doing that worked for him quite well."

Tom: "I know what you mean. I've thought several times that I should try to look upon discomfort and pain as just the current roll of the dice. I enjoyed good health and had many wonderful days, which I accepted thoughtlessly, only thanking God now and then. If my lot is now to suffer from bad health and have to endure some bad days, well, that's the way it is, and I should accept that from God also. I don't think I should say that pain and suffering are good, something that God enjoys handing out. But I do think I should try to accept them and ask God to make my acceptance of them something useful."

John: "I couldn't put it better. We should never call obvious evils, physical or moral or social, something good, merely because by enduring them people can be made holy. But we should try to accept the mysterious fact that God has made a world in which such evils exist, trusting that somehow God can justify the way he has chosen to create us."

Tom: "Do you think God has complete say in the matter? How directly is God responsible for my pain? The other day somebody was telling me about a book he'd read that pictured God as limited, maybe even helpless, granted the random character of the universe God has made."

John: "Boy, that's a complicated, tough question. There has been a movement in the past twenty years or so to speak that way, because the random, complicated character of the universe and evolution has started to make an impact on theologians. But something deep in me resists such a move. First, I think it fails to own up to the mysteriousness of God, which includes the possibility that God, in the divine infinity, can do all sorts of things we cannot understand and has all sorts of operational modes we cannot fathom. Of course theologians have to do the best they can and are bound to use human categories when trying to understand God. But sometimes they seem to get far removed from the primordial wonder that contact with the living God is bound to generate. Sometimes they act as though they could spin out rules, theorems, that God would have to obey. Everything in me says that's nonsense. God is always the measure, never the measured. Second, I think that God has to be present to everything that exists, and that without such a presence of God there is only nothingness, non-being. One can do a tap dance and show that evil is a disorder and so non-being, but that's an apologetic suitable only for a few intellectuals. For the many common people (and maybe for all the suffering people), the only apologetic I find adequate is Christ's cross. On Christ's cross God dealt with pain not by explaining or justifying it but by embracing it and using it to bring forth a new creation. On Christ's cross God fulfilled the promise given to Moses at the burning bush and made the divine nature known to those who would sojourn with him. Our covenant has always been with a mysterious, hidden God whose name we never know. What we learn about God comes from traveling and wrestling with God. For Jesus that meant ending up on the cross, and if we truly believe that Jesus is the divine Word become flesh, then *God* suffered and died on the cross. In other words, the nature of God includes God's embracing the suffering and death that are our worst nightmares. That's the sort of response to pain that most justifies God in my view. There's nothing we can undergo that God himself hasn't experienced directly, at first hand. I hope that, when my time to suffer and die comes, I can cling to this fact and find it a sufficient 'explanation.' "

Tom: "Is that right—*God* died on the cross? How can God die? Don't you mean that the man Jesus, who represented God in a special way, died in trust that God would receive him?"

John: "Getting quite theological in your old age, aren't you? Well, I meant exactly what I said, though what you said is also true. Jesus, who was fully human, died on the cross, the way that any of us human beings would die if we were strung up. But who was Jesus? Yes, he was a specific individual, a Jew of the first century, the son of Mary and Joseph, and so forth. But Christians have confessed for more than nineteen centuries that the inmost reality of Jesus was more than human, was in fact divine. How that could be so is a profound mystery, but unless that is so the entire cult of Jesus—worship of Jesus, in the strict sense of *latria,* the cult one may offer only to God, on pain of otherwise being an idolater—that Christians have practiced throughout their history has been a dreadful mistake or sham. So the affirmation of the divinity of Jesus is crucially important. One may admit that explaining or clarifying the divinity of the man Jesus is an enormously difficult, in a real sense an impossible, task. But there it stands, in the creeds and the liturgies and the convictions of the saints. Two further things. From early times the conviction was that unless Jesus had been divine (unless it was the divine Word who had taken flesh from Mary) human beings were not saved. Only God can save us, in the sense of making us so whole that we become partakers of God's own immortal existence. So if Jesus were only an expression of God, a man whom God inspired, a special saint, then salvation did not occur definitively. Second, because of the union of the divine and human aspects of Jesus (because of their both being predicable of the same subject) we can say that divinity, God the Son, was the 'personal' reality, the subject, of the death of Christ on the cross. That does not mean that the divine Son ceased to be or expired. But it does mean, in all proper obscurity, that at the depths of his human personality the Jesus who died was the divine Word, even in his dying. The technical term for this theological usage is 'the communication of idioms,' by which is meant the legitimacy of applying human attributes to the Word and divine attributes to the humanity of Jesus, because of the unity of Jesus the God-man."

Tom: "You seem quite exercised about all of that. Why is it so important to you?"

John: "Because salvation is so important. Without a definitive accomplishment of salvation, which Christians traditionally have believed Jesus accomplished by living, dying, and rising as he did, our hopes for a complete justice, fulfillment, success for the whole venture of creation are unfounded. Critics of the Christian conviction about such a definitive salvation sometimes say either that it shows an immaturity (wishful thinking) or that there is no reason to prefer Christian salvation to what one can find in Hinduism, Buddhism, or some other religious reality. Let's not get into the question of comparing religions, unless we have to. It's very complicated. But, sticking just to Christian tradition and culture, let's make it very clear that if one depicts God as helpless in the face of creation and history, then creation and history are absurd, in the literal etymological sense of offering nothing for us to 'hear,' giving forth no meaning. It's one thing to claim, on supposedly empirical or rational grounds, that this in fact is exactly what one finds in creation and history: no obvious meaning, no comprehensive sense. It's another thing to describe oneself as a Christian and admit such a claim. To my mind you can't put the two entities (Christian faith and no definitive salvation) together without heresy—deformation of Christian faith. In the measure that I find Christian faith more precious than anything else in the human repertoire for exploring reality and living well (wisely, creatively, realistically, lovingly), I think I'm bound to hate the deformation of Christian faith that twists it out of shape and suggests that it's impotent or a fraud—not what Jesus himself promised not what from earliest times Jesus was understood to have accomplished."

৯৯

Tom: "Tell me again how this relates to my pain."

John: "It relates to your pain quite directly: God found a way to experience what human beings go through when they suffer and die. God went into the jaws of death, let them close around him, and emerged in a way that made death penultimate ever after. This is perhaps the sharpest angle of the stumbling block that the goodness of God presents to us. We find it nearly incredible that God should have defeated death and opened for us vistas of literally unending, eternal life. But that's what Christian faith says, and that's why those who want to water down Christian faith seem to me pernicious dwarfs."

Tom: "I don't know. You seem to be saying that because God has accepted pain, suffering, and death into the divine existence they have been changed once and for all. I'd like to believe that, but I don't experience pain that way. The pain I've had to endure has rendered me unable to think or pray well, if at all. It's been nearly completely negative."

John: "God forbid that I start to give you lectures on the significance of pain, when you are suffering and I'm standing here indecently healthy. Your pain is what it is, and what you experience it to be has to be what you offer to God, however mute or implicit such an offer has to be. What I have to say about pain is only as legitimate as the detached speculation we sometimes fall into late at night, if we have received a decent theological education and the cognac has done its job. Nonetheless, I believe there is valid place for such speculation, inasmuch as part of our human vocation is to try to make sense of our experience and faith. But such speculation never can substitute for the actual endurance of pain that we're called upon to accomplish. It's not those who work out a clear picture of the redemption of pain but those who manage to endure who enter the kingdom of heaven."

Tom: "Don't be so apologetic about speculation. The ideas you've given me have been precious in a way you probably can't understand. Where I was nearly completely inarticulate, you, or the Christian tradition you're telling me about, have given me words, ways of naming my experiences, my doubts, my fears, my hopes. Naming them, and so making them things I can reason and pray about, has helped me to tame them. Certainly, my fears remain in part wild beasts, things I'll probably never tame, but simply by correlating them with the experiences of Jesus I've been able to exorcise much of their demonic character."

John: "Thanks for telling me that. It's good to hear. And, as I think about it, it relates to the anger you saw flare up in me a few minutes ago. I grew up furious at the small-town culture of the Massachusetts suburb in which I lived, because it pretended to catalogue all people and assign us our places, from which we weren't suppose to move. In the case of my family, we lived in the wrong end of town, went to the wrong church, came from a somewhat undesirable ethnic background, and, most pertinently, were stigmatized as the family of an alcoholic—an obvious failure. The fact that nose-in-the-air people from uptown were making these judgments, as I knew instinctively they were, whether they realized it or not, set my blood boiling, because I was positive all their judgments were utter crap. My father was a wonderful man, much more loving and struggling than most of those prissy, superior types could even think of becoming. So when I realized that faith offered a completely different view of human beings, one much less categorical and much more mysterious, I sensed in my bones that I wanted my whole life to be immersed in that different view, that appreciation of the mysteries and paradoxes of life which alone could render either God or real, live human beings their due. I remember stopping physically in the middle of the street—I must have been about ten years old—and realizing, in utter clarity, that I need not be the victim of other people's judgments, or even of my own fears, because I could *think* about things: get distance, perspective, realism, and so control and freedom. I was exorcising my demons, which I would now say were the fear that human existence was haphazard, absurd, exactly as the nose-in-the-air self-important types professed it to be, by their arrogant dismissal of what I knew in my bones: people like my father, and the family of us so shaped by his weaknesses, are claims on God for a justice and meaning the world never gives."

Tom: "I don't know what to say. You seem on the brink of something very exciting yet very difficult."

John: "It's probably more heat than light. But maybe it explains a little why I find those who apparently play around with faith and skepticism so despicable. A pyschologist might say that I'm simply defending mechanisms I found necessary for coping with pain when I was young. I would grant that entirely, but rejoin that all of us who are honest, or have enough depth to merit the name adults, have had to grapple with such pain. If so, then those who deny the significance of our grappling and the mechanisms, including most prominently the religious faith, we've found viable are the enemy, both ours and God's, because they reject the very essence of the human struggle, trying to laugh it away. Where we human beings have been made to wrest meaning from our pains and joys alike, they cop out by fixating on money, or status, or clever distraction, justifying themselves by saying there's no meaning to be gotten. To be charitable, one probably should say that they do this because they cannot bear to look their own demons straight in the eye. Distraction and trivialization have become their coping mechanisms, carrying the pathos of despair. But they are so influential in the academic circles in which I move that I find myself despising them. I think it would be bearable, were they to say, in humility and honesty, that they don't know where to find meaning in the universe or their own lives, that their experience and best struggles to date have not shown them a clear path. That would be unobjectionable, even admirable—something I'd have to accept, even feel compassion for, though I continued to think or wish that a better exegesis of their experience would show them potentially wonderful meaning. But when they are haughty, arrogant, dismissive, when they try to rule meaning, religion, commitment to creativity and love out of court as adolescent or unsophisticated; then my gorge rises as it did forty years ago, when I stopped abruptly in the middle of the road and realized I need not be the prisoner of the phony s.o.b.'s who were trying to relegate me and my family to the margins of significance, trying to make us losers and no-accounts so they could feel superior. As I say, in a more charitable mood I can find myself reaching out to the faithless secularist and thinking that the more arrogant he or she appears the more trouble or pain probably lurks below the surface. But on the level of existential argument, where one's views are one's self, I find those who deny the redemption of our pain and call people looking for redemption naive truly repulsive, dangerous human beings. And you should too, because they imply that what you are going through is just hard cheese, your bad luck. It has no meaning and you're not going to be any better for it, even if you endure it heroically. Meanwhile, they will shake their heads, pretend to commiserate, and not so subtly patronize you, in the name of some superiority their good health apparently confers on them."

ॐ

Tom: "There's a sort of kindness that comes over me now and then that sweeps away the anger you describe. Or maybe it's just that I'm used to most of my acquaintances dividing into two camps, one so completely secular that the question of over-all meaning never gets raised and the other so biblically pious that the question never has any teeth to it, having been decided from the outset. If I were to get angry at those who seem to deny the significance of the struggle in which I'm engaged, I'd have no rest. I *know* that I've got to make sense of this cancer and the death it brings closer every day. I'm *sure* that the grounds I find for hoping it will not all have been a dreadful waste, an exercise in futility, are precious beyond rubies, when they hold up and don't seem contrived. The metaphysical impli-cations of either the defeatism of most people I meet or my own conviction that they have to be wrong are beyond my compe-tence, and so beyond my interest. What I want are ideas, analy-ses of actual experience, that hold up in the light of day, when I can be relatively rational, and that don't let me down in the dark of night, when I can feel overwhelmed. There *has* to be mean-ing, a plan, a redemption of failure and pain. I'm as sure of that as I am of our need to eat or sleep or find love. If many people want to call my conviction a defense mechanism or wishful thinking, that's their problem. Until they have come into a limit-situation such as mine, I'm not inclined to give their opin-ions much weight. And even if some of them have come into limit-situations, are facing death or outright evil, I'm still not inclined to pay defeatism or nihilism much heed. It doesn't fit either my own experience or what I take to be the testimony of the great sages and saints, so it's as easy to dismiss as the piffle one sees in the tabloids at the checkout counter of the super-market. There Elvis has been sighted in Nevada stepping out of a UFO or a huge woman is screaming that she ate her baby while sleep-walking, because of the fad diet she had been following."

John: "Yes, the checkout counter spotlights the dregs of popular American culture. I'm amazed, though, that you are so strong in your convictions about the necessity of life making sense. I don't want to embarrass you, but that strikes me as an eloquent testimony to the work of the Holy Spirit in you. We attribute to the Holy Spirit the strengthening of faith, hope, and love that enables us to defeat infidelity, despair, and selfishness. Have you thought about the presence of God in your conviction and determination?"

Tom: "No, not in those terms. I have been surprised, at times, to find myself tightening my jaws and getting very firm with myself, and sometimes with the people around me, determined that this death of mine is going to be as 'good' as I can make it. But I sense that these are still early days, when it's easy to gather up my will. I don't know how I'll fare when weakness threatens to become listlessness, lassitude, or when pain makes me raw. The doctors say they will be able to control most of the pain, but I don't want to lose lucidity until I absolutely have to. I'd rather be uncomfortable than lost in narcotic journeys, off in other worlds."

John: "Let me offer you something I read years ago—I can't remember where, perhaps a saying of the French theologian Henri de Lubac. The gist of it was that when we suffer with grace or ease, we're not really suffering. Pain only conforms us to the cross of Christ when it makes us ugly, defeated, reduced to a vestige of our pride and achievement. I think maybe the author was glossing the idea that the suffering servant was so reduced to such misery. Let me see whether I can find it here in your Bible. Isaiah 53:2–3: 'He had no form or comeliness that we should look at him, and no beauty that we should desire him. He was despised and rejected by men; a man of sorrows, and acquainted with grief, and as one from whom men hid their faces he was despised, and we esteemed him not.' Isaiah probably had in mind the reduction and despoliation of Israel during the exile to Babylon. The followers of Jesus quickly cast Jesus' sufferings on Calvary in the lineaments of this suffering servant. Either way, the biblical message seems to be that life can reduce any people, including the people of God, as both Jews and Christians have liked to call themselves, to something with no dignity or beauty. The ravagements of evil, whether physical evil such as cancer or moral evil such as the holocaust, can break us and make us pitiable. Yet that is not the last word. It was not the last word about Israel, whom Isaiah was convinced God somehow would restore. It was not the last word for Jesus, whom his followers convinced God raised from the dead in complete triumph. And we can struggle to believe, on such warrants, that it need not be the last word here and now, for us. But I would not underestimate the act of surrender that may be required of us: to let go of consciousness, dignity, even the last shreds of self-control, hoping against hope that these violations will somehow turn out to have been the final takeover of a wonderful lover. That's how some of the most impressive saints seem to talk: God will make their death the consummation of the love affair he has been pursuing with them since they first drew breath."

Tom: "You're right on the mark about the worst horrors: losing control, dignity, ability to function significantly as a human being. I find the loss of attractiveness easy enough, perhaps because I've never thought of myself as any movie star. That can be handled with a joke or a wry shrug. But to be so preoccupied by one's pain that one can't think well, or pray, or pay any attention to other people, or appreciate the grass glistening after the rain—that's hard to handle. I guess I am like most westerners in locating my self in my mind and will, my sense of autonomy and self-control. We all know that death takes that away, but the kinds of death that take it away slowly, agonizingly, are especially repulsive."

John: "Yes. It's instructive that virtually all pre-modern peoples have surrounded death with taboos, even though they have frequently dealt with it more straightforwardly than we do, not sequestering the dying away in cul-de-sacs. For most pre-moderns, death and blood made one unfit for religious activity, for consorting with the divinities, because they put one out of phase, rendered one alien. Pre-modern thought was more complicated than that, of course, but this aspect of it still suggests the horror native to the human spirit when it is forced to contemplate the often ugly breakup of its world, the so proximate threat of the dissolution of the body which has been the only housing it's known. I've sometimes thought that the aging of America that we're now witnessing has been changing the face of death, and perhaps for the worse. To see the pictures, or visit and get the first-hand reality, of the people warehoused in facilities for the very old can seem to be to witness the elongation of death, its expansion into an extended process. Certainly some very old people accomplish marvelous spiritual feats from time to time and perhaps redeem their situation. But I've been thinking that a good death would be neither premature nor overdue, and that a good death is a consummation devoutly to be wished and prayed for."

Tom: "I agree, very much. My own death is premature, I suppose, though not by too many years. I've sometimes consoled myself by thinking that it could be worse to be dying ten years beyond the male norm, rather than ten years before. And such thinking has raised the question of euthanasia. What do you think about that? Should we start to lift our absolute prohibitions against helping the moribund hasten their death? I know you have to go now, but promise me we'll talk about that next time. Watching other patients on this ward, even more than thinking about my own future, has made euthanasia a real question."

§◠

Tom: "Remember your promise to say something about euthanasia. The more I think about dying pitiably or uselessly, the more the question lures me in."

John: "Another difficult issue. I guess there are no easy issues, where pain and death are concerned. First, I have to say that I believe that Christian instinct leaves death mainly in God's hands. There are qualifications or exceptions, of course, but the foundational feeling, it seems to me, is that because we did not create life we have no right to destroy life or end it before its apparently natural time. What then about war and capital punishment? Any justification for them comes from the fact that the enemy or the criminal has forfeited some rights, through unjust and dangerous behavior. For the sake of the greater good, one can go to war against an unjust aggressor or remove from the community a person who broke its code of conduct heinously. Does suicide or euthanasia fall into the same category as war or capital punishment? Only by some tortured analogies. Suicide implies that one can take over the process God has in mind for one's death. Euthanasia implies that an outsider can abet or effect a suicide. (If someone professing to be accomplishing euthanasia were not carrying out the patient's will to die, the project would be simply murder.) So, I believe that people who confess the dominion of God over their lives have to have a negative reaction to suicide and euthanasia."

Tom: "But don't we challenge or supplant the 'dominion' of God in dozens of ways: intruding into the biosphere, manufacturing artificial limbs, practicing birth control, and on and on."

John: "Certainly, so the question becomes whether hastening death is parallel with interventions that we don't usually consider assaults on God's dominion (though of course the propriety of all three of the interventions you mention is debated and in none of them would I grant human beings absolute dominion). I think death is significantly different, because it is final. Admittedly, my view depends on a balance between God's creation of a human life and God's ending of that life. People who put the beginning of human life into human beings' hands, finding conception and ensoulment to have nothing gratuitous about them, can easily say that we should be able to end what we begin. That doesn't square with my instincts, though. I think that both the creation of life and its ending at death are so mysterious as to be holy, things we ought to reverence and intrude upon only with great care."

Tom: "Does your position require people to hang on endlessly, sustained by respirators long after their brains have died?"

John: "By no means. I think we have little obligation to take extraordinary means to prolong life once it has clearly reached its 'natural' term. People can debate what 'natural' means, but to my mind once a person is diseased and would die if machines did not take over key bodily functions, death is at hand and perhaps it should be allowed to take its course. So I'm saying that we should neither hasten nor retard the time when, as much as we can judge such things, God wants to end a life and take the person to himself."

Tom: "I guess the lawyer in me wants something more precise than that. How can we defend doctors and hospitals against the charge that they have terminated life prematurely by not supplying means that would have prolonged it? Theoretically God could work a miracle and restore the person's intellectual capacities, justifying our having kept him or her on a respirator."

John: "With all due respect to the legal profession, I think that lawyers and insurance people have complicated medical care beyond any rightful influence they should have on it. In the process, they have made legal liability and money far too important. The fear of malpractice suits now wields an influence clearly inordinate. People need defenses against incompetence, but there is no way to build an error-free world, whether in the hospital or outside of it. At some point we have to accept the fact that we live in an imperfect world, especially regarding its social dimensions. At some point we have to call such imperfection God's will. Where that point is in a given case can only be decided on the spot, prudentially. But just as we have to accept the fact that cars and planes are going to entail lethal accidents, so we have to accept the fact that some deaths are going to occur sooner than we would like. If we believe that God is capable of redeeming all death and injustice, we should be ready to let people die when reputable medical opinion and common sense say their bodies dictate."

Tom: "How much weight do you give to the quality of life people are able to manage near the end? At what point does the pain or mental incompetence of people so take away their quality of life and dignity that it would be a mercy to end their lives?"

John: "I can't say, and I don't think anyone else who believes in God's presence in people's lives can say either. Once again, the example of Jesus is instructive. God did not spare Jesus the diminishment of the quality of his life and dignity entailed in his crucifixion and death. Obviously, the correlation between Jesus, suffering in the prime of life, and a terminally ill cancer patient is not exact. Yet the instinct of Jesus to bow to God's will, God's way of letting things work out, and commending himself into God's hands seems to me entirely relevant. Difficult, in some ways superhuman, as this may be to grasp ahead of time, I think that when people of faith actually encounter God's will that they suffer and die they can find it consoling to accept that will and commend themselves to whatever God has in store for them."

Tom: "But doesn't that run the risk of fatalism? How can one know what is God's will and what is something we ought to fight against? For example, would you limit chemotherapy or radiation to cases where there was at least a fifty percent chance of remission?"

John: "I don't know, Tom. I'm not pretending to have certain wisdom about all this. I guess I think there are some cases where it's clear one ought to fight and take every reasonable measure—for example, if the person is relatively young, or has special responsibilities (the parent of young children leaps to mind), or has a special work underway, or even just feels a great anger against the cancer and a great love of life and so passionately *wants* to fight. There are other cases in which age, the virulence or spread of the disease, the person's sense of not having the will to fight, of wanting the disease just to take its course, or of wanting to avoid the troubles of chemotherapy could overweigh the obligations to fight. It's the kind of decision so personal and existential that there's considerable leeway for the individual's discernment of what in fact God seems to be moving him or her to want to do. Our moral principles only carry us so far. Frequently there's still a gray area we have to clarify for ourselves, ideally through prayer, good counsel, and courageous reflection. I can see two different people faced with roughly the same circumstances coming out with two different answers and both of them being right. Life is not an absolute good and death is not an absolute evil. The main good to be sought, I believe, is what seems to be God's disposition of us, God's will. I think God generally wants us to love life and defend it, but that God also wants us to accept death, when it's appropriate. There's nothing simple about living with God. Each day we have to search for the divine presence and try to attune ourselves to the divine will. Once again, look at the way that Jesus lived and died. Much was evolving and variable, but at the core of Jesus' teaching and behavior alike lay the will of his Father, which served him as a true north by which he could set his compass."

Tom: "So you're opposed to euthanasia, though not simplemindedly."

John: "I hope not simplemindedly. The difficult question of the costs attending people's longer living today adds another wrinkle, but my instinct is that if we were to avoid special interventions in the cases of the elderly and moribund we could eliminate many such costs and honor the right of people to die when their bodies dictated. Of course what interventions are 'special' and how the body 'dictates' the time of death are freighted questions. But we can never eliminate the need for common sense, and good doctors and clergy ought to be able to help both the elderly themselves and the people concerned with their care to bring such common sense to clarity."

4

Wisdom

Tom: "I've been thinking that we can correlate the caution you feel about euthanasia with a general principle to the effect that there are wisdoms our bodies may perceive earlier or better than our minds. Granted, the interaction between mind and body is intricate and mysterious. Sometimes I've felt I should simply follow the lead my body seemed to be providing, and sometimes I've felt I had to reject my body's apparent advice. In the question of migraine headaches, for instance, my experience has been that there are times to fight the onset of an episode and times to give in and let it take its course."

John: "My experience exactly. The same with whether to push oneself when one is feeling tired or give in and say the body is telling one it's time to take a break."

Tom: "Applied to the course of a disease such as cancer, though, such a wisdom becomes both more pressing and more difficult. For example, what happens to the natural 'voice' of the body when it has been medicated significantly? Unless one reverts to a position that rejects all drugs and medical interventions, the advice the body wants to give may be altered, even contradicted, by the changes introduced by the treatments to which it is subjected. Nonetheless, I keep listening to my body, hoping it will tip me off about how things are progressing inside of me and what mental attitudes I ought to take. At the least this is an interesting game, and sometimes I think I've been helped by it."

John: "Tell me what your body has been teaching you about the invasion of death. Does your body report incursions by a resented stranger, an enemy, or does it seem benumbed, fatalistic?"

Tom: "Probably both. The bleeding that first took me to the doctor for tests raised some alarm, but there was no pain so the problem was to control the wild fantasies to which my imagination could run. I went to the first surgery thinking that the entire situation—diagnosis and likely prognosis—was unreal, because it had not manifested itself in gross ways, other than the bleeding. I had not suffered any significant decline in energy, and I was just beginning to notice a loss in weight. The pain from the first surgery brought a quantum leap in my perception of the reality of the situation. What graphs and charts and test results could render only abstractly the bodily pain made extremely concrete. Still, there was the question of distinguishing between the pain of the cure (the operation) and the pain of the cancer. Now that I'm starting to experience a general deterioration, the lesson of the fatality of my disease seems to be coming in a twofold mode. On the one hand, I'm feeling more fatigued, though some of that may be psychological. On the other hand, I'm starting to accept the evidence of general breakdown and so no longer am expecting or hoping for signs of improvement. Combined, these two factors may be teaching me that I have to begin to detach myself from life as I've known it to date, including the bonds with other people that I've forged, enjoyed, and used to help me determine who I am."

John: "Let's talk about both of these factors, and then about such detachment. Tell me more about what you are making of the weakness you're starting to feel."

Tom: "It's both disturbing and pacifying. I resent losing my appetite for food and work, conversation and future prospects. Yet something about being pushed to let go of these things, to attend to the deeper question of what is happening to me, which in turn asks me to decide who I want to be at my end, is appealing, if frightening. I remember from my freshman philosophy course that Plato spoke of the love of wisdom as the practice of dying. I hadn't thought of that for forty years but it popped up the other day, no doubt because I needed it. Anyway, so far much of my reaction to the physical invasion of the disease has been like what one experiences with the flu. Because there has not been great pain, it's been a question of going with the flow of what takes your strength, so that you're willing to surrender yourself to sleep or rest."

John: "And the fading of your expectations or hopes that you might get better—that the next report might be encouraging, that there might be something positive to anticipate?"

Tom: "Yes, that's been instructive. At first it was depressing, but now I take a strange comfort in the inevitability of my decline. I guess you could say I've stopped kicking against the goad. Also, I've noticed a pull to shift my hopes to another direction, which perhaps says that we're bound to keep hoping, right to the end. Since the tests and physical prospects don't hold much promise, I've started to think about placing my hopes in God. Not for a miraculous cure. After a few forays in that direction soon after my diagnosis, I haven't thought much about miracles. But for an embrace of God, or an embrace by God, that would give me firm ground, while all the physical grounds for hope are crumbling. I guess I want to rest my spirit in something as incontrovertible, and unprovable, as God's promises to stand by us, to be kind to us right to the end."

John: "Is the detachment you mentioned just another side

of this shift of your hope to the mysterious supports God may offer?"

Tom: "At bottom it may well be, but on the surface my detachment is fairly stoic. I want to be realistic about what is virtually certain to happen to me. I want to deal with my family, the doctors, my friends, the people with whom I am finishing up details of business, and everyone else straightforwardly, putting right on the table the prospects I do and don't have. I don't know why this has become so important to me. One reason, in all likelihood, is the experience I've had of dealing with dying people, and perhaps even more with their families, where the cards didn't seem to be on the table. I have found that very awkward, unhealthy even, and in recoil no doubt have decided to go to the other extreme. Another reason is that the people who have done the most for me, throughout my life in general and concerning this question of how to deal with death in particular, have been the straight shooters. I've admired them very much, especially when they did not flinch from admitting, and operating in view of, the hard truths, the disagreeable realities. If there is any good example or edification I would like to give others in my dying, it would be to persuade them that honesty is the best policy right to the end."

John: "I don't know why, but there just flashed in my mind the saying of Confucius that by the time he had become seventy he could do whatever he wanted, because his will and the dictates of the Tao (the way of virtue he found laid out by the ancient Chinese sages) had become one. You speak as though honesty had become a physical need."

Tom: "Exactly. I need to be honest, or at least to try to be honest, as much as I need to feed my body and my mind. Being honest, in fact, seems to take the modality of feeding my spirit, giving its hunger for truth and realism its due. It has always bothered me to have to ignore glaring realities or chatter about insubstantial things. Now most of the social pressures to conspire to keep harsh realities out of sight have fallen away, though not all of them, so I can be more forceful about insisting on honesty and concentrating on what is really important."

John: "I want to hear about how it works out when you try to concentrate on what is really important, but first fill out your remark about the social pressures not to deal with harsh realities, especially the pressures that have not abated."

Tom: "Well, people who visit me exhibit the general unease with cancer and death that afflicts our culture at large. And of course I can understand this, since I've often felt it when dealing with sick people or their families. We can get into an awkward, though somewhat amusing, situation in which I am sensitive to their sensitivity to my sensitivity to the topic of my death. I try to cut through all of this by giving them a frank report about where things now stand and then talking about the lessons I've been learning from my illness. Some of my visitors handle this reaction quite well, but others blanch and are soon gone. Too bad, but I have no stomach for playing games of false cheer, so I don't mind their leaving."

❧

Tom: "About detachment, my main thoughts have been circling around our insignificance, in the total scheme of things. When you consider how long the universe has been in existence, or the millions of years through which mammals have evolved, or the nearly incredible distances between the stars, you have to scale down the importance of your own situation, and that can be comforting. I've come to the same conclusion by considering the profusion of human lives: over five billion of us now and God knows how many billions more throughout human history. Each of these lives has been mortal. Each has entailed pain and, we can hope, joy. There must be little in my life that qualifies as unique or special. So I shouldn't make a great fuss about my losses and regrets. I'd do better to appreci-- ate the grandeur of the cosmic scheme in which I've been privi- leged to play a tiny part. It helps my spirit to concentrate on that, saying 'Thank you' to the creator who gave me my chance."

John: "What you say reminds me of the whole problem of egocentricity. Psychologically, we miss a great deal of reality, and burden ourselves with many pains we could avoid, by as- suming that we are the center of the universe. As a species, we stay blind to the havoc we're wreaking on the environment long after the facts have been plain because we think cosmic history pivots on *homo sapiens.* I suspect some of the relief you derive from thinking about the bigger, truer picture is another benefit from realism. Just as realism can seem to nourish our spirits, teaching us that we're made to live in the truth, so it can seem to lift great burdens, teaching us that illusion is a heavy weight, a great oppressor."

Tom: "I expected you to contradict my arguments for insig- nificance, reminding me that the New Testament says that God numbers all the hairs of our heads. Are you telling me that my detachment admits of a Christian interpretation?"

John: "I guess so. First, and preliminary, is the notion that any genuine truth has to be referable to God, since both truth and God are one. Second, there is the idea that grace, God's self-communication, is everywhere. Whenever anyone pene- trates the truth or casts off illusion, Christians ought to suspect the movement of the Holy Spirit. Third, why do you think that the detachment you sketch is incompatible with God's provi- dential care? Couldn't God be leading you to just this detachment?"

Tom: "Well, my ideas don't make much provision for a personal God, and I haven't known how to correlate this sense of resignation or submission to a bigger picture, one that puts egocentricity or anthropocentricity in the shade, with surrender to a personal God."

John: "One of the main lessons taught by mystics such as John of the Cross, who report on what it's like to experience the touch of God directly, is that they are weaned from false perceptions and consolations, sometimes painfully. God forces them to detach themselves from the idols, the self-concerns, the ambitions that have kept their worlds tiny. If they are going to be capable of sustaining intercourse with the real God, who is completely sovereign and beyond human imagining, as well as completely loving, they have to be stripped of their illusions and cleansed of their sins, most of which boil down to self-centeredness. So, it seems to me quite congenial to speak of God's personal care for an individual leading that individual out of self-centeredness and into a much better appreciation of the objective vastness of the universe. I don't think that vastness contradicts the possibility of each individual creature, especially each rational creature, having an immense significance."

Tom: "But how can each rational creature have an immense significance, when there are so many of us, and we all die, and the universe is so much greater than all of us put together, to say nothing of any particular one of us?"

John: "Because God is not limited the way we are, and so God does not suffer the overload that vast quantities bring to us or the depletion of qualitative responses, such as love, that we suffer when we try to extend our range. There is no contradiction between God's having made billions of us, and our span being much less than that of the stars or the seas, and God's caring passionately for each of us, even to the extent of involving himself in a love affair with each of our hearts. The same God who hurled the stars into their places, as the Bible might picture it, is the one who St. Augustine was convinced is 'more intimate to me than I am to myself.' Paradoxically enough, when we start shedding our anthropocentrisms we find that our imaginations can expand, so that we are less likely to put limits to what God can do than we were when unaware we were making human spirituality the limit of what God can be or do. Nothing that is not a self-contradiction is impossible to God, because God is the source, the font, of all possibility. And though one might reason to most of this philosophically, the better warrant for such a view, in my opinion, is the way that Jesus depicts God. Not a sparrow falls without God's awareness and interest. Consider the lilies of the field, how they grow."

Tom: "But don't the two sets of feelings diverge? Isn't the emotional atmosphere of the detachment I mentioned, cool and resigned, quite different from the warmth and attachment one associates with the speech about the lilies of the field, the prodigal son, and the like?"

John: "The feelings are different, perhaps divergent, but that doesn't mean they are incompatible. All of our feelings about God as well as our ideas, are but paltry little tools for investigating a vast reality and possibility we shall never even begin to appreciate. The foolishness of those who think heaven will be boring becomes clear when one catches a glimpse of how much there is to know and love about God. It is literally endless. God never stops, so appreciating God need never stop. Take your most creative moments. Haven't they shown you further possibilities unfolding to the point where they receded from your imaginary sight? Well, God has to unfold like that, has to be a treasure-trove or thesaurus of beauty and intelligibility and power and love that we could never exhaust. In that treasure-trove there must be goods and deeds that elicit the cool, detached feelings you've suggested, the ones created by an awareness of how vast God's universe is and how much in it is impersonal. On the other hand, there must also be in the treasure-trove goods and deeds of God that elicit a warm, passionate love and interpersonal appreciation. There I would place the history of salvation, centered in the sacrificial love of Christ displayed on the cross. One might join the two sets of feelings by reflecting that the one who suffered on the cross was the divinity we have been hymning as unlimited, stretching to the ends of the galaxies and the depths of the subatomic particles. The being that exists at these extremes is referable to the intelligibility of the godhead itself, which Christians traditionally associate with the Word, the divine 'person' who became flesh and experienced human existence in the identity of Jesus of Nazareth. Actually, then, Christian speculation about providence, the way God cares for the world and is present to the world, becomes immersed in trinitarian theology, much to the surprise if not despair of some eighteenth century Christian apologists, who wanted to keep the whole business away from what they considered irrational or provincial beliefs such as the Trinity. Perhaps that's how you feel, too."

Tom: "No, it's not that I'm opposed to the Trinity. It's just that I've never known how to think about it. It's always been presented as the most arcane of the mysteries, the realm of the high flyers. Better for the likes of me to concentrate on more accessible and experiential matters."

John: "I see. One of the tragedies of church life nowadays is the unfamiliarity of ordinary members, and not only ordinary members, with the wellsprings of Christian tradition. The theologians bear a heavy burden for not having translated into contemporary language such central matters as the Trinity, the incarnation, and grace. Those are the mainsprings of Christian faith, the cardinal doctrines, not papal infallibility or the governmental structure of the church. Yet the peripheral matters get ten times the attention the cardinal doctrines do, to the great detriment of Christian vitality. If the core doctrinal symbols mean little to the average Christian, the spiritual life—reflection, prayer, understanding of mission—is bound to suffer. Presumably the key symbols bear most directly on the mystery of

God, otherwise they would not be key: up front in all the classical creeds. To neglect the key symbols therefore is to impoverish people's dealings with the mystery of God. Naturally, God is not limited by human folly, so God continues to deal with people in their depths. But the impact of God's dealings, at least when it comes to such outward matters as teaching and shaping culture, is blunted because the exegeses of religious experience that the tradition has deemed most profound suffer great neglect."

Tom: "Tell me why the Trinity is so important. What difference could better appreciating the Father, Son, and Spirit make in my preparation for death?"

John: "Quite a direct challenge. Ok, you're on. Consider this: the most telling name for God in traditional eastern Christianity was *athanatos*—the deathless one. In contrast to human beings, whose most salient feature was their mortality, the divinity was deathless, immortal, and so dramatically other. This instinct lay deep in classical Greek culture, so when Greek culture became Christianized it loved to contemplate the deathlessness of God. As the traditional Byzantine chant about God puts it, 'Holy God, Holy Mighty, Holy Immortal, have mercy on us.' Those words 'holy,' 'mighty,' and 'immortal' have all carried a powerful resonance. Not only do they name the mystery at the center of Christian prayer, the Father to whom all prayer ascends, they also name the community into which faith takes the devoted Christian at death. Faith itself is a process of immortalizing, of divinization: becoming sharers of the divine nature. As early as Plato, in fact, Greek thought had spoken of the human vocation as 'to become as much like God as possible.' No wonder that the Greek church made Plato virtually an elder statesman, comparable to the biblical prophets and evangelists."

Tom: "And the relevance of this to either the Trinity or my preparations for death?"

John: "Sorry, I was digressing. The relevance lies in the riches of the godhead suggested by the symbolism of the Trinity. When it came to describing the life of the deathless God in which Christians began to participate through faith and upon which they hoped to enter in fulfilling measure after death, the fathers of the church, developing hints in scripture, sketched something communal. Starting with the usage of Jesus, as he appeared in the gospels, the fathers had two key names for God, Father and Spirit. Eventually they decided that these three—Father, Jesus (the Logos incarnate), and Spirit—named something identical with the one God revered by the Jews, Jesus's people and the spiritual progenitors of the church, yet also something more differentiated. 'Differentiated' is my word, not theirs, but I think it names the fathers' conviction accurately. In using the names Father, Son, and Spirit, the church believed it was articulating a clearer understanding of the divine mystery than had been possible before the revelation communicated in the person and teaching of Jesus. True, the Hebrew Bible had spoken of the 'Word' of the Lord and his 'Spirit.' The Christian trinitarian language therefore had precedent and could be considered somewhat traditional. But the Christians intuited an advance in appreciating the inner life of God. The Father was the biblical Lord not only personalized in an especially intimate way but more clearly set in relation with a self-expression and lover, the Son. And the Spirit somehow indicated a process related to the relation of the Father and the Son that communicated their mutual love. So one might say that without wanting to postulate three divinities the early Christians opted for a communitarian notion of God. Monotheism in the sense of a featureless self-sufficiency was not the richest appreciation of the divine Lord, the creator, the love that moved the stars (to jump ahead to Dante's phrase)."

Tom: "Let me see if I'm with you. The Trinity names a sharing within God, a relationality (if there is such a word), suggesting that communion, connection, is as primordial, perhaps more primordial, than independent being, autonomy."

John: "Very good indeed. That philosophy major would have made you as good a theologian as a lawyer. All of this is stuttering, of course, but still profitable. When great minds such as Augustine and Aquinas stuttered, the 'image of God' long dear to patristic usage, due to its meditations about the status of human creation, became precisely an image of the Trinity. Then, taking such human faculties as memory, intellect, and will as their favorite probes, such theologians spoke of the Trinity as an infinite fullness of awareness, understanding, self-expression, mutuality, and love. For Augustine, the Father was a recession without end, an unbegotten beginning, like the backreach of the amazing human faculty of memory. For Aquinas the Father was a blazing act of understanding, an insight without limit, totally comprehensive. The Son, for both, was the expression of the Father, different from the Father only because begotten, not unbegotten (the expression, not the expressor). The Spirit was the love generated by the mutual knowledge of Father and Son, a love that circled through all of their communion. Together, Father, Son, and Spirit inhered in one another, forming a perfect and completely unlimited community of light, life, and love. Their mutual inherence, which did not destroy the 'order' of their relationships, secured their unity, so there was no danger of thinking of them as three gods. But their relational diversity, the difference they had as Father and Son, or Father and Spirit, or Son and Spirit, gave a richer picture of their oneness as the single godhead than would have obtained without Jesus' revelation of the divine Fatherhood, Sonship, and Spirituality."

Tom: "Is any of this experiential, or is it all merely speculative?"

John: "Well, 'experiential' is a tricky word, because the things we believe—the names we use, the conceptions we instinctively employ, even the speculations that color our explorations of the external world and our reflective talks with ourselves, as individuals or in groups—are ingredients in what we call experience. Experience is not brute or unformed. The more we bring to an encounter, the more we tend to find in it, the more it can register in us. So, if we pray as Christians schooled in trinitarian imagery and concepts, we are more likely to think we are moved by the Spirit, or brought toward the Father, or stand alongside the Son than we would be if we came to prayer with no such imagery and concepts. Still, the thrust of your question remains: What practical difference does trinitarian theology make, perhaps especially in view of death? The first thing that comes to mind, right now, is that the imagery of the Trinity shows us something of the 'inside' of God, and that as such it represents a self-disclosure of God, accomplished in Christ, that should be very consoling. You know the saying of Jesus that he has not called us servants but friends, because he has revealed to us the things in his heart (as friends tend to do to friends, but masters seldom do to servants). Well, the main things in Jesus' heart were his relations with God. The treasure of his life was his relation with his Father, which dominated his sense of his mission: to reveal the Father and serve the Father's will to save all humankind. The mystery of Jesus clearly reposed in his being led by the Spirit, who after his death would be for Jesus' followers the same sort of 'helper' that Jesus himself had been. And the depths of Jesus' own identity lay in the Logos, the eternal Word spoken by the Father that had assumed flesh from Mary. When we contemplate the God into whose hands we commend our spirits at death, these images of what lodged in Jesus' heart should cheer us greatly. We are going to an encounter that Jesus has prepared: pioneered, prefigured, and secured in success. We are going home, to a richer familial existence than we could ever have expected or hoped. And our family, our home, is the perfect unity-in-diversity of the divine persons."

ॐ

Tom: "I'm intrigued by the notion that diversity-in-unity, or community, may be more primordial than oneness. It challenges the individualism of modern western thought. I also like the idea of joining a divine family, a fullness of life based on sharing."

John: "Parallel to the way that we have neglected the trinitarian imagery for God, we have also neglected the trinitarian imagery for the relations with God that we summarize in the word 'grace.' Since God remains one, the same, whether subsisting alone or engaging in relations with creatures, it is the trinitarian God who dwells in our hearts and moves us to all that is good in our lives. What heaven, 'glory,' will consummate and make definitive has already begun in grace: intimate sharing with Father, Son, and Spirit. The Johannine literature of the New Testament makes it plain that loving Jesus takes his followers into the relations with the Father and the Spirit that structured Jesus' life. Those who abide in the love of Jesus deal with the Father, perhaps under the modality of the limitless creativity, resourcefulness, power, and possibility that intercourse with the divine spirituality can suggest. They also deal with the Son, perhaps under the modality of gaining confidence that the world is grounded in an intelligible plan and human beings can go out to the mysterious source of the world (the Father) confidently, like children sure they will be well received. And those abiding in the love of Jesus perhaps deal with the Spirit, sent by Jesus and the Father, under the modality of the force that settles them in this faith-filled interpretation of the mysterious depths of themselves and creation. The Spirit is God given to us and received, welcomed, in our hearts. It takes more faith and imagination than I have to make this trinitarian interpretation of what goes on in the depths of the human spirit predominant in one's sense of the ultimate significance of daily living, but from time to time it emerges into consciousness to remind me that I'm in way over my head. My boat is very small indeed, and the ocean of divinity has more treasures than I shall ever comprehend. What holds me in being is the paramount force in creation, far more powerful than evil and death. Otherwise, evil and death would be the first and last word, which clearly they are not."

Tom: "Even if one were to experience one's depths, where the mind runs into darkness and the heart can only try to pray wordlessly, along the lines of the trinitarian modalities you mention, God would still remain incomprehensible, would he not?"

John: "Absolutely. The Trinity may be a more differentiated symbolism for God, but what it articulates and colors still remains infinite and so beyond anything in us human beings: mind, heart, emotion, or imagination."

Tom: "So the practical import for someone like me, praying in face of death, would be more reasons to trust, hope, and appreciate the goodness of God, rather than my having to clarify doctrinal issues and find them sufficiently congenial to confess. 'Faith,' as you have been describing it, is more an acceptance and trust of the God pointed to by the creedal symbols than something preoccupied with those symbols or articles themselves."

John: "Certainly. And faith always is dealing with a God bound to defeat our symbols, even those most privileged symbols we call creedal or biblical. God is more unlike than like our assertions about God, even when our assertions are completely true, inspired by God, and precious because orienting us rightly toward the beginning and beyond of our existence. We never know what God is. The most we get are hints, glimmers, analogies, similes that we can trust, because of Jesus, the church, those who have preceded us in faith. They have received a language about God and the life that responds adequately to God's love that did not let them down. They received it from the divine mystery, they believed, and it enabled them both to live for God, in service and witness, and to die trusting in God, full of hope that God would take them to himself. The consolation of dying in continuity with this tradition is that one is following so admirable a cloud of witnesses. But not even this cloud of witnesses can remove the darkness and mystery of the whole venture. Nothing can substitute for God. Only God can represent God accurately, fully, adequately, which is why the Holy Spirit has to be the final maker of one's prayer, the final carrier of the dying into the Father's embrace."

Tom: "It boggles the mind to think that divinity itself is the inmost reality of one's being and faith, and that death is the way we become freed to plunge into divinity, lose and find ourselves in divinity as we never could while alive in the flesh."

John: "It certainly does. From a dozen different angles, the storehouse of Christian wisdom says that we can never overappreciate the significance of God in our being, our lives, our selves. God is the source of everything positive in us. God is the one toward whom our spirits reach, in every longing to know or love, every incremental gain of knowledge and love. The revealed symbols we take from the Bible, which pivot around Christ, embellish all this, so that all of our needs and hopes become ways of expressing what God probably is doing on our behalf and wants us to become. And, frightfully yet wonderfully, we never get surety about any of this. God never comes under our control. The surety God offers lies on the plane of love, not knowledge. If we ask God for bread, is it conceivable that we will get back a stone? If we, evil as we are, know how to give good things to our children, will not God give us all that God has to give, all that we want purified and pressed down, so that our cup runs over? That is the logic of faith, 'justifying' a reliance on God in trust. That is the 'reasonable' defense one can advance for offering God carte blanche."

Tom: "You've moved the trinitarian language back to its more homey origins in the teaching stories of Jesus. It seems less speculative and more easily grasped there. I can follow the logic of trying to deal with God as Jesus did, like a child trusting in an utterly good parent. I can see why the women in our church have been talking about calling God our mother, as well as our father: the one to whom we go in trust could as well be the one who gave us birth as the one who directed us lovingly. And, somewhat to my surprise, the idea of becoming like a small child, in order to enter the kingdom of this parental God, does not put me off. If serious illness does anything, it teaches you your vulnerability and smallness. Sometimes humorously, sometimes depressingly, you learn that you're not the master of your own fate. Others take you where you don't want to go—other forces, other purposes. The most powerful of these are beyond your ken: the cancer, the aging, the dying. You can only hope that they will turn out to be bread, not stones—dispositions of a good God. So maybe a major function of death, a major reason God has built it into the life-cycle, is to clarify what have always been the true proportions of the relations between us and God. We are the pots, not the potter. We didn't make ourselves, so it's not surprising we don't control our mode of dying. In fact, I've been thinking about how many things were never under my control, even when I had full health and thought I was at the top of my game. Is it T.S. Eliot who speaks of our passion being more profound than our action? Dying certainly makes that obvious, and I'd like to think that all along God has been the prime mover. I only wish that I had been more aware and responsive, better at seconding God's initiatives, or at least appreciating the mysteriousness of the game in which I've been involved."

5

Love

Tom: "I think our discussions have brought me to love theology, for the first time. The ideas we've been exchanging, and the reading I've been doing, have been exciting, nourishing, consoling far beyond anything I ever expected. It's as though for years I longed to discuss what faith actually could mean, how God actually could be working in my life, in our world, but I didn't have the time, or the vocabulary, or the desperate stimulus necessary to satisfy this longing."

John: "Well, you're pretty remarkable. I can't think of many other people, healthy or ill, with whom I've been able to pursue fresh inquiries into what the creedal symbols have to say about our actual lives, in their depth and mystery, their confusion and promise and pain."

Tom: "Oh I don't know. I may be unusual in having had the education, or the speculative inclination, to wrestle with the new ideas—new to me—that you and I have been discussing. But I suspect that many people brought into a situation like mine want to make sense of what's happening to them. How many would find biblical or traditionally theological language congenial, I can't say, but I'm quite sure that many have the problems, the questions, the needs that the biblical and traditional language was coined to handle."

John: "Tell me about the love of theology, or better the love of the divine mystery that inspires theology, that you have found."

Tom: "I'll tell you what I can. On one level, it's clear even to me that a big draw is the consolation Christian faith and theology offer. The more I muse about the traditional symbols and ideas, the more I understand why they have been called 'good news.' It doesn't bother me that many sophisticates dismiss them as antiquated wish-fulfillment. Cancer makes you quite free of the opinion of sophisticates. You've no more need to kowtow to the fashions of secular intellectuals than to the fashions of Pierre Cardin or Ralph Lauren. It's so clear that you need words to live by, reasons to hope, that all the brittle chatter of the sophisticates makes little impression. 'Put them in my position,' you're tempted to say, 'and see how their nihilism plays.' On a second level—one that I hope is more significant to me—I've come to love the peace that pondering the implications of faith regularly has brought. Sometimes I only read or think for a few minutes before I don't want any more. What I have taken in seems so rich that I just want to chew it over, asking God to help me believe it, to rivet it into my soul, so that I can accept what is happening to me and be grateful for the opportunities I've had, including the opportunity to prepare for my death and discover in it possibilities I'd never dreamed of."

John: "How does that sort of pondering make God appear to you? Are you finding yourself more able to love the divine mysteriousness?"

Tom: "Yes, oh yes. It's not clear to me where the mysteriousness of my own life, spotlighted by the breakdown of my body and the uncertainties surrounding death, ends and the mysteriousness of God begins, but my suspicion is that the two overlap. If God is more intimate to me than I am to myself, as I have it on your authority that Augustine says, then what I might call the human mystery overlaps with, or is concentric with, or—probably better—recedes into the divine mystery. Once I accepted the notion that 'mystery' doesn't mean a puzzle so much as a too-fullness of significance, a plenum too rich for a finite intelligence, I began to see mystery everywhere: in the endless expanses of the galaxies, in the amazing complexities of the human body, in the creativity of the human mind, in the intricacies and wonders of human love, in the darkness surrounding our being. To push on any fact, any idea, any emotion has been to move closer toward mysteriousness, and gradually it has become clear that mystery is the primary phenomenon while our clarities, our facts and conclusions and sure projects, are secondary. I've come to sense the 'ecological' character of both human existence and the universe: how everything is related, and how the ground of the whole network of relationships is mystery in a comprehensive sense."

John: "And this mystery has become lovable?"

Tom: "Not always. Sometimes it has been threatening. I can't get my mind around it, and when I forget that no one can, that we're not supposed to be able to, I'm unsettled. Other times the mystery has had no resonance for me. I've been too tired, or worried, or strung out, or something. But enough times the mystery has seemed sufficiently pregnant, alluring, supportive, richly textured (like black velvet) to buoy me up and make my heart go out to it in love. Why should there be such a variance in the faces the mystery presents, or the receptions I've been able to give it?"

John: "I don't know, but it's the common testimony of people who try to deal with God regularly that sometimes they are consoled and sometimes they are flat, even depressed. In the middle, which means the majority of times, they are somewhat attracted yet feel they are struggling—overmatched, not up to the challenge of appreciating God as they ought. Most of the classical writers on prayer suggest that one can only try to perse- vere, trusting that God has good purposes for this swing of moods and experiences. In general, the good purpose such writers spotlight is our purification—the deepening of our real- ization of who and what God is, in contrast to who and what we are."

Tom: "Who and what are we?"

John: "In this context, face to face with the living God, we are quite imperfect creatures: 'sinners,' in a word. Our consola- tion should be that God accepts us despite all our imperfec- tions, and our gamble should be that whatever God does to us, in us, is an expression of that acceptance—an act of love de- signed to help us grow and prosper. Obviously, often that is hard to believe."

Tom: "Yes, but I've found it remarkable, astounding, to read the gospels with an eye sharpened by need and see the love of God that Jesus teaches. On the other hand, I've also found it sobering to see the demands that Jesus makes in the name of his God and to confront the theme of judgment. I guess what has preoccupied me is the conjunction of these two themes. Love and judgment, even condemnation, both weave their way through the gospels. If you tore out either one you'd unravel the entire fabric. Can you really say that all of the judgments of God are expressions of the divine love? What about God's punish- ment of sinners?"

John: "I find that a very complicated question, specula- tively, and something I tend to ignore. I've made the determina- tion, or the choice, that the love of God is more fundamental, or central, or important than his judgment, so I interpret judg- ment in terms of love, rather than vice versa. In other words, I've given more weight to parables such as that of the prodigal son than to stories such as that of Dives and Lazarus. I've leaned on John and Paul to make the synoptic Christ one full of the divine love, so that his sharp tongue is peppery rather than fully angry and his power to handle demons or to work cures is controlled by his concern for the needy people at hand. One of my biggest problems in reading the New Testament is not being able to see the expression of Jesus' face as he speaks or acts, and not being able to hear the tones he uses. So much interpersonal meaning is conveyed by our looks, gestures, accents, body language that having only the bare text is like working blind. From the general drift of the Christian proclamation, its overall self-presentation as good news, I've fashioned what one might call a hermeneutic of kindness. That is, I assume that Jesus is usually taken with people rather than put off by them. Though they try his patience, it is easy for them to win his heart. Any expression of honesty, need, faith, love not only gets his attention but secures his sympathy. That's the interpretative gamble I've made. I think it has good grounds, but not everyone makes it as I do, and by the time I've extended it into a full theology, where I find myself saying that in all his dealings with us God is only loving, I realize that I'm way out on a limb, trying to face down not only the fears in my own psyche but also the ravages of history and the waste one finds in nature, the carnage and pain. Still, what else can I conclude, if I love more than anything the evangelical thought that if even we, evil as we are, know how and usually want to give good things to our children, God must be wanting to be good toward us beyond anything we can appreciate? So while I admit the judgment scenes, even the imagery of the divine wrath, I make that secondary, believing and hoping that it is merely another way of conveying how serious God is about the offer he's made to humankind. Because that offer has been an act of love, it's had to trade in the coin of freedom, which has meant that human beings could really reject God. The judgments of God, I believe, are merely God's acceptance of self-condemnations that people unwilling to respond to God's love have worked already. Scripture portrays God as angry, or, perhaps better, heart-sore, because of the rejection of his love and the waste, the ruin, that ensues."

৯৯

Tom: "Several times I've felt well up in me a poignant love for the beauty of human life. The physical world, the people I love, the body that has served me so well until recently—all have seemed so precious they've taken my breath away. The prospect of losing them has been very painful, yet along with that emotional pain has come an analgesic of gratitude. Realizing that they were always only on loan to me, as gifts of God, has helped put my loss of them in perspective. But the tears running down my cheeks have amazed me. One day my favorite nurse came in and started to cry with me, as a reflex, I guess. I couldn't explain to her why I was crying, and why there was more joy than sorrow in my tears. She had the good sense simply to hug me, and I thought afterward of all the things I've embraced through my life. Certainly the most precious has been tender human flesh, and that's where most of the regret and love focus. The hardest thing is to think of leaving those who have become flesh of your flesh and bone of your bone. I know that this process of dying is detaching me from the many different things I've loved, but to date it hasn't removed my delight in the people I've cherished, and I hope it never does."

John: "I hope so too. The incarnational character of Christian faith seems to make it different from the many other religious faiths that urge detachment from material things, or indeed from any objects of desire. No doubt the priority of God implies that we should have some detachment from lesser goods, but the incarnation of God's Word qualifies such detachment. To the end Jesus seems to have loved his life, the world, the people around him. The stories of his dealings with the good thief and the apostle John from the cross suggest this. When Jesus commended his spirit into his Father's hands, I suspect that all that he loved went with him. He was giving to the Father the entirety of himself, and that must have included all those he loved. When Paul elaborates the union between Christ and his followers so that they comprise one body with him, this inclusion gets full expression. Christian faith intuits there is a symbiosis between Christ and his followers, a common life. We can hope, therefore, that all we love will go with us when we pass over to God. We can hope that our family and friends will be with us in heaven. That is the implication of the creedal article about the 'communion of saints.' Just as the inner life of divinity itself is communal, so the life of creatures with God is communal. The one hundred and forty-four thousand that the book of Revelation places in heaven praising God are symbolic of the myriads we hope will greet us when we enter upon the beatifying vision of God."

Tom: "I've noticed that it's almost a regular method with you to take the experience I've described and run it through a sort of theological transformer. It comes out elevated, purified, raised up so I can see its richest potential. Is that deliberate on your part?"

John: "No, but it may well be instinctive. I believe that theology has always sprung from experience and that it only comes alive when it is illumining experience. Interesting as it may be to move the mind along the tracks of pure logic, so that one can reason out the implications of certain propositions, that soon begins to pall. Theology is not mathematics. Its subject matter is intrinsically mysterious, and, as Christian, theology is incarnational. So it only achieves its full resonance when it has become '*faith* seeking understanding.' Specifically, it only achieves its full resonance as Christian theology when it stays in close touch with the flesh of Christ. That flesh makes Christian theology intimately sacramental and metaphorical. It speaks best, in my view, when it speaks poetically, so that it evokes the mysteriousness of the incarnation. Consequently, I instinctively tend to grab onto a handful of experience, such as your narrative about the poignant love of human flesh that has welled up in you recently, and try to reconfigure it in terms of the leading metaphors of Christian faith. The metaphors, to say nothing of all their interconnections, are so rich that I never know where I'm going to end up, but the ride is always profitable."

Tom: "I suspect that sacramentality doesn't mean as much to me as it should. You've linked it to the incarnational character of Christian faith. How would this apply to human mortality?"

John: "Two applications come to mind immediately. The first is the sacrament for the sick. In praying with the sick and anointing them with holy oil (a traditional sign of God's blessing and the 'seal' of the Holy Spirit), we try to bring our faith in God's saving love to bear on the crisis, the special moment, facing the sick person. All the sacraments admit of interpretation as symbolic rituals designed to mediate faith to especially significant occasions. The hope with final anointing is that both the body and the spirit may benefit from prayer, community support, the laying on of hands, and, above all, the advent of the Holy Spirit, our most profound comforter. The traditional wisdom here is very physical, and so less suspect than other approaches might be. It deals with the actual situation gently but straightforwardly, with no avoidance. In that way, it links up with both the honesty that has been so important to you throughout this trial and the love of the mortal body you are having to give up. The second thing that comes to mind is the eschatological motif present in eucharistic theology. Eschatology, as you know, is concerned with the last things, the finalities and endings of Christian existence. For the central Christian sacrament, the one whose basic symbolism is the nourishment of divine life in us, to carry powerful overtones of immortality is quite striking."

Tom: "The relevance of the sacrament of anointing, as you describe it, is easy to see, and very consoling, but I'm not sure I follow you about the immortality of the eucharist."

John: "Let me find the most relevant biblical passage in your Bible. I know that it's from John 6. Ah, here it is. Jesus said, 'Truly, truly, I say to you, unless you eat the flesh of the Son of man and drink his blood, you have no life in you; he who eats my flesh and drinks my blood has eternal life, and I will raise him up at the last day. For my flesh is food indeed, and my blood is drink indeed. He who eats my flesh and drinks my blood abides in me, and I in him. As the living Father sent me, and I live because of the Father, so he who eats me will live because of me. This is the bread which came down from heaven, not such as the fathers ate and died; he who eats this bread will live forever.' "

Tom: "Explain, professor. I recognize the plain sense, which is hard to accept, but I suspect there is more going on."

John: "There's almost always much more going on in John's gospel—it's so deep and symbolic, so rich with irony and allusion to prior biblical themes. Our time is running out, so let me just sketch some of the main points, with the promise that I'll return to them tomorrow. First, Jesus is disputing with his opponents, who refuse to accept him as a divine emissary. Second, in the background is the miracle of the multiplication of the loaves and fishes, when he fed the crowd physically. Third, Jesus is playing off the symbolism of manna in the wilderness, when God fed Israel through its wanderings. The implication is that what was only prefigured there is being fulfilled here, in the presence, the person, the flesh of Jesus himself. Fourth, there is the theme of divine life. God is the only one who lives death-lessly, so to gain eternal life one must participate in God. Jesus is saying that by eucharistic communion, by eating the bread and wine that represent his flesh, his followers can indeed participate in divine life. Fifth, to underscore that it is Jesus' flesh and blood that people eat is to recall his death, when his blood was shed and his flesh was sundered. The bread broken and the wine poured out recall that death. Receiving them, the believer has Jesus abide in him or her, which means that the believer abides in Jesus in return. Such abiding is the quintessence of the Johannine view of grace: participating in divine life, through communion with Jesus, the personal 'place' where divine life became most incarnate and so physically most available in history. By communion with Jesus, mutual abiding with him, one communes with the Father and Spirit as well. The Johannine literature is the richest New Testament resource for the correlation of grace, incarnation, and the Trinity. Since that correlation is the backbone of Christian doctrine, orthodoxy always owes a great debt to the Johannine writings."

 formats

Tom: "You were going to continue to relate eucharistic theology to sickness and death."

John: "Yes. Not to be prolix about it, let me simply say that the 'life' so central in the Johannine view of God and the eucharist is the antidote to sickness and death, and that that life is identical with the love and light characteristic of the Johannine God. What Jesus reveals is the comprehensive beauty, power, and efficacy of God, whom he calls his Father. To accept Jesus by faith, commune with him through the eucharist, and abide in his love is to receive at one and the same time the light necessary to dispel sinful ignorance, the life necessary and sufficient to overcome sin and death, and the love that is both our best indication of what God is like and the fulfillment for which we've been made. All of this radiates from both Jesus himself and the eucharistic sacrament through which believers commune with Jesus. All of it also radiates from the Johannine Spirit given by Jesus to secure his followers in the light, life, and love that he shares with the Father and the Spirit."

Tom: "That vision seems more positive than the Pauline view of the struggle between sin and grace."

John: "I think perhaps it is, though with a different logic Paul reaches many of the same conclusions. For John the key moment in the history of salvation is the incarnation, when the Word takes flesh. By God's coming that deeply into the human condition, the human condition is radically changed. For Paul the key moment is the passover of Jesus from death to resurrection. Paul likens that to a new creation. But the effect is the same for both writers. The life that believers share with Jesus the Christ defeats sin and death, on its way to entering the new phase called 'resurrection.' "

Tom: "So the wages of faithful abiding in Christ and communing with him through the eucharist are resurrected life, in contrast to the wages of sin, which are death."

John: "Yes. That's a good mixing of the two theologies, the Johannine and the Pauline."

Tom: "What are the proportions of individualism and universality in this mixture? How much is resurrection, as a symbol of the triumph of Christ and his followers, applicable to the whole world, as well as to individual believers?"

John: "That's difficult to say, but it's clear that both Paul and John think cosmically. The Logos is the power holding the entire world together, giving the whole of creation its intelligibility. And the 'world,' in the sense of the sinful realm opposed to God's grace, is defeated by the triumph of Christ. I used to think that these symbols were too abstract to be helpful when it came to thinking about the massive problems of poverty, pollution, injustice, and the like, but over the years I have changed my mind. For over the years it's become clearer that our great problems are interconnected. If you read the reflections of theologians working in Latin America, where the grinding poverty and the constant carnage threaten to blight every day, you find them speaking about original sin with a specificity that nails it right to the examining board. They have become aware of the systemic character of disorder and sin on their continent. Poverty and death are not accidental. They tend to occur inevitably, because of the economic and political arrangements that have grown up. So one has to contemplate tearing up the entire network of twisted relationships among money, power, cultural pride, ideology, and the like, if one wants to conceive of an education, health care, economics, and religion that would produce different effects. We in North America have our own equivalents of the twisted systems that have devastated Latin America, epitomized perhaps by the homeless people in Washington living across from the White House. Even more troubling, though, is the evidence that poverty everywhere is in part the result of economic and political systems that have now become global. Equally, the environmental pollution that now threatens virtually all countries is in significant part the result of these same systems. So to speak of a power stronger than the 'sin of the world,' than the systemic disorder rooted in human folly and greed, is to speak of a grace poured out for all of creation. In fact, it is to speak of a divine life, an intimate presence of God, capable of overcoming the twistedness that rebel creatures have created. My view, therefore, is that the individual is merely a microcosm of the overall global patterns, and that it doesn't take much reflection to realize that all of us are pushed out of shape by vicious structural injustices."

Tom: "Are you saying, then, that when I contemplate my own situation any solution Christian faith may offer in fact applies to the comprehensive problem of a world sick unto death from sin?"

John: "The hands are those of Tom Carney, but the voice is that of Søren Kierkegaard—I catch the reference. Yes, certainly. There are no gimmicks in the spiritual life, the life of our struggle for faith, hope, and love. That's why, in an important sense, there is no special doctrine or pastoral practice for the dying. Your situation clarifies the great need that people always experience. You need ways to believe that life is stronger than death, that love is more powerful than hate. You need to connect yourself with such life and love, if you are to feel confident that your death is not the last word. What C.S. Lewis called 'mere Christianity' is the only response I can offer you. Nothing else is so radical and comprehensive. One of the signs of our weakness and sin is our tendency to run away to fashionable alternatives —humanistic psychology, for example. Certainly there is wisdom in many such alternatives, but most are mute in face of death and systemic evil. The best they can offer is a graceful stoicism. At the other extreme, one finds the lunatic fringe that expects science or the spiritual power of a supposed 'new age' to change creation. They would have us freeze our corpses in expectation of a twenty-first century technology that could cure the cancer or heart disease that had killed us. I think most of the current western alternatives to the radical analysis and cure implied in the gospels are pitifully superficial. Think again about the promises expressed in that part of the eucharistic discourse of the Johannine Jesus that I read. Think about living forever by abiding in Christ. It's no surprise that people's minds boggle and scamper away to find less demanding visions. The permanent scandal of Jesus is the claim that he experienced eternal, resurrecting life, and that he shares it with those who commune with him."

Tom: "You're back to the theme that the gospel is not too strange to be believed but too good."

John: "Yes. We find it hard to face either the depth of our need, our sin, or the still greater, the literally inexhaustible, depth of God's response, God's goodness."

Tom: "Ok. The obvious question is: Why isn't this goodness more manifest in the world? How can one speak of salvation when so much manifestly is unsaved? I have had a fortunate life, so my terminal illness is only a petty tragedy. But the majority of human beings throughout history have been scarred by terrible suffering. If Jesus has saved the world, why has there been all this suffering? Why does it continue today?"

John: "Let me deal with that tomorrow, please. You look tired, and I don't want to take away energy you need for your family. You've been so strong in dealing with them that they've come to depend on finding you relatively composed. I promise I won't avoid your question, though I have to warn you that there's not a very satisfactory answer. But right now let's just place the whole thing in God's keeping, ok? 'Sufficient for the day is the evil thereof.' Like the devil, I can quote scripture whenever it eases my getaway. See you tomorrow."

ॐ

John: "When we talk about the reality or unreality of salvation, we ought to speak concretely. For example, we ought to begin with what we have experienced at firsthand. I have to say that goodness has outweighed evil in my experience, and that the evils I've seen or been forced to contemplate have been tamed by the possibilities faith has held out that God's love still could be greater. The light has kept shining in the darkness, and the darkness has not been able to overcome it. It's not my place to say whether everyone else, or anyone else, can or should be able to make a similar confession. Similarly, it's not the place of the atheist or the Buddhist to speak for others. We each have to speak for ourselves. Having spoken for ourselves, we certainly have the right and duty to think about how goodness and evil, salvation and the lack of salvation, seem to be faring in the rest of the world, or seem to have fared in past history. But in exercising this right and duty we should retain a proper modesty. Not being able to speak from the inside, from actual experience, about what other people are experiencing or what happened in past centuries, we ought to put cautions, hedges, around all our judgments. Christian teaching that God gives all people sufficient grace for salvation. I take that to mean that God gives all people help sufficient to enable them to feel grateful for the good things that happen to them and not succumb to despair because of the evil things. But how such grace actually operates in people's hearts, how they experience or think they fail to experience God's love, is not mine to say. It isn't anyone's to say. Each life is a mystery even to the person living it. Ultimately we all have to *believe* that our time has been worthwhile. We shall never have definitive proof that we have used our time well enough to stand justified before our creator. We can never be sure on empirical grounds that God was wise to have made creation as God in fact did. We all have to hope that we have aided the light more than the darkness and been worth the love God bestowed on us, the extravagant love revealed in Christ."

Tom: "So you're saying that it's presumptuous of me to ask about the efficacy of salvation, at least in the sense of wanting empirical arguments that more people have found their time in the sun good than have found it bad."

John: "Yes, I guess I am. I'm also saying that each of us ought primarily to attend to ourselves and the portion of history over which we have some influence. God won't ask us whether we were able to justify God's ways in the world. God rather will ask us how we used the graces we received, the love lavished upon us, and whether we made it easier for those we encountered to believe in the worthwhileness of their lives."

Tom: "So the entire business of salvation is a mystery from beginning to the end."

John: "Exactly. It's bound to be, because it all depends on God, whom we can never grasp."

Tom: "Why is it that that answer is so, so . . . so I don't know what: maddening, satisfying, frustrating, amusing? I want to punch it, all the while that I'm touched by it, that I laugh about it, that I find it more realistic than any alternative I've ever met."

John: "God has a great sense of humor. Often I find myself straining to hear echoes of a heavenly laughter. Our condemnation to mystery would seem cruel, except for the motif that the mystery stretches us toward maximum growth. What kind of a plan of salvation—what kind of a God, if you come down to it—would it be if we could understand it? How profound or beautiful or loving could Jesus have been, if his human audiences weren't puzzled, intrigued, delighted, and scandalized at being confronted with something beyond them? There's a certain infinity in us, a certain limitlessness of reach and hope, and the mysteriousness of what we glimpse of the divine plan matches up with this infinity, delighting us. But our infinity is housed in a very finite container, so we also want certitudes, clear and distinct ideas. God did his best to let us have it both ways by enfleshing the divine mystery. Jesus made the mystery as close and objective as flesh that people could touch, a voice that people could hear. Yet God could not make divinity unmysterious, simply factual, because that would have been to misrepresent how God actually is, and so would not show me the truth that, as Jesus said, sets us free. So God seems to smile in wry amusement, as the people of God, the children of God, fuss and stew and finally realize that love and laughter take them much farther than demands, or irritations, or flights, or rejections—all the ways people can refuse to accept the most obvious fact about our human condition: we don't know, we have to believe."

Tom: "So we should place our money on Jesus and love, if indeed we can say that Jesus is the best revealer of the divine mystery we have found and that love is the most precious of our human experiences."

John: "That's the way I think the wager falls out for the Christian. One can make it ever tidier: we bet that the love associated with Jesus—the love he shows in the gospels and the love we experience when we consort with him—is the pearl of great price, the great treasure for which we ought to be willing to sell all we have."

Tom: "I would like to be able to say that I've lived for such love, for such a God. I would like to have been such a witness to that love that others would have found it attractive. The best I can say, though, in echo of Augustine, is 'Late have I loved Thee.' "

John: "We all have to say that. That's another wrinkle of the mystery. What in times of grace seems so obvious has been obscure most of our lives. We haven't lived by the obvious fact that we can't understand our situation and so must let mystery have its way with us. We haven't followed through on our intuition that Jesus is the revelation of God, the enfleshment of the divine mystery, given us to light our way. We have forgotten, compromised, procrastinated. We have been unprofitable servants, sometimes in the extreme. Yet the message is that God nevertheless has always loved us, has never stopped loving us, has never given up on us. The foundation of our hope, then, is not ourselves. The foundation is God himself. In another of the numberless divine mercies, God has not let us, who are so limited and fragile, be the measure even of our own significance.

Our lives have been hidden with Christ in God. We shall only learn the real significance of our lives when we meet God in the risen Christ who sits at God's right hand."

Tom: "Will you pray for me, that I meet God that way?"

John: "Of course. Many of us have been praying for you all along."

Tom: "I know. Sometimes I've felt your support, almost physically. I'd also like your blessing. I know you're not in the blessing business, but you believe in it, don't you?"

John: "I do. There's a lot of peasant in me yet. The Lord bless you and keep you, Thomas Carney. The Lord make his face to shine upon you and be gracious to you. The Lord lift up his countenance and give you his peace. May Almighty God bless you, Father, Son, and Holy Spirit. May he send his angels to guide you to his paradise, so you can meet the Son who died for you and feel to the full the love poured out upon you from the foundations of the world."

Tom: "Thank you—for everything."

John: "No, thank you. You've helped me far more than I could ever help you. I'll see you soon."